GREEN SMOOTHIE REVOLUTION

GREEN SMOOTHIE REVOLUTION

The Radical Leap Towards Natural Health

VICTORIA BOUTENKO

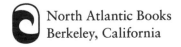

North Atlantic Books
Berkeley, California

PUBLISHED BY
North Atlantic Books
P.O. Box 1232
Berkeley, California 94712

COVER AND INTERIOR PHOTOS: Robert Petetit
PHOTO OF GABRIELLE CHAVEZ ON P. 21: Julia Corbett
COVER AND BOOK DESIGN: Claudia Smelser
Printed in the United States of America

Disclaimer: The information contained in this book is not intended as medical advice. Victoria Boutenko does not recommend cooked foods or standard medical practices. The authors, publishers, and/or distributors will not assume responsibility for any adverse consequences resulting from adopting the lifestyle described herein.

Green Smoothie Revolution: The Radical Leap Towards Natural Health is sponsored by the Society for the Study of Native Arts and Sciences, a nonprofit educational corporation whose goals are to develop an educational and cross-cultural perspective linking various scientific, social, and artistic fields; to nurture a holistic view of arts, sciences, humanities, and healing; and to publish and distribute literature on the relationship of mind, body, and nature.

North Atlantic Books' publications are available through most bookstores. For further information, call 800-733-3000 or visit our website at www.northatlanticbooks.com.

LIBRARY OF CONGRESS CATALOGING-IN-PUBLICATION DATA

Boutenko, Victoria.
Green smoothie revolution : the radical leap towards natural health / by Victoria Boutenko.
      p. cm.
   Includes bibliographical references and index.
   ISBN 978-1-55643-812-7 (alk. paper)
   1. Nutrition. 2. Smoothies (Beverages) 3. Cookery (Greens)
I. Title.
   RA784.B639 2009
   641.8'7—dc22
                                        2009005069

    1 2 3 4 5 6 7 8 9 United 14 13 12 11 10 09

To my children,
Stephan, Sergei, and Valya

CONTENTS

PREFACE The Green Smoothie Revolution Has Begun   ix

PART ONE UNLEASHING THE HEALING POWER OF GREENS

1 The Miracle of Greens   3
2 Greens, the Key Ingredient in Human Nutrition   7
3 The First Green Smoothie   15
4 The Importance of Rotating Greens in Your Smoothies   21
5 Blending versus Juicing   27
6 A Green Smoothie Q&A   31
7 Green Smoothies for Our Children   37
8 Green Smoothies for Our Pets   41
9 Food Combining in Green Smoothies   45
10 Guidelines for Optimal Green Smoothie Consumption   47

PART TWO GREEN SMOOTHIE RECIPES

Valuable Tips and Tricks for Smoothie Preparation   53
Green Smoothies for Beginners   57
Supergreen Smoothies   73
Savory Green Smoothies and Soups   81
Green Smoothies for Adventurous Souls   99
Green Puddings   107
Green Smoothies for Children   119
Green Smoothies for Pets   127
Green Smoothies for Body Care   129

AFTERWORD The Worldwide Green Smoothie Revolution   131
APPENDIX 1 Amazing Weight Loss: A Case Study   135
APPENDIX 2 Clent Manich: Living on Green Smoothies   143
APPENDIX 3 How the Raw Family Went Raw   151
INDEX   159
ACKNOWLEDGMENTS   173

PREFACE
THE GREEN SMOOTHIE REVOLUTION HAS BEGUN

THE GREEN SMOOTHIE REVOLUTION IS HAPPENING NOW, THROUGH you and me and everybody else in the world who is enjoying this delicious green drink. The most stunning fact about this magic potion is that while it is supergreen in color and extremely healthy, it is also delicious beyond anyone's expectations and is easy to like. In my classes and workshops I have watched thousands of people undergo a profound transformation when they try a green smoothie for the first time. Their disgust and trepidation about the "green stuff" suddenly turns to delight at the smoothie's surprisingly delicious taste. I inevitably hear an audible "Wow!" and watch people licking their cups clean.

Having spent fifteen years trying to inspire people to incorporate fresh fruits and vegetables into their daily diets, I remember how hard it used to be to convince others to eat more raw food. For many years I drove eight hundred miles along the West Coast teaching weekly classes about raw food. I taught a ten-week course in cities from San Francisco to Seattle. Then, after a week's break at the end of a course, I would start all over again. Despite my colossal efforts, the majority of my students found it challenging to maintain a raw food diet.

That situation has radically changed with the arrival of the green smoothie. Ever since I put together the very first green smoothie in August 2004, the drink rapidly started gaining popularity without much promotion on my part. Today, more people are aware of green smoothies than of a raw food diet. I can now order a variety of green smoothies at several of my local juice bars, and even at the drive-through near the airport in Medford, Oregon. Many TV shows and magazines are endorsing green smoothies, and when my children recently took me to the movies, I almost fell off my seat as I watched Iron Man pull out a blender and proceed to make a green smoothie.

Ever since the invention of the green smoothie, I have been drinking them daily and sharing them with others. I love green smoothies so much that I am committed to drinking them until the last day of my life. Everyone in my family fell in love with them, and many of our friends did too. Wherever I go, I gather new information from green smoothie fans worldwide. Through everyday blending, research, and letters from our readers, we have compiled the best recipes and basic principles of green smoothie creation and consumption in this new book.

I hope you enjoy discovering the world of green smoothies, and finding your favorite recipes for optimum health. Happy blending!

—*Victoria Boutenko*

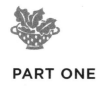

PART ONE

UNLEASHING THE HEALING POWER OF GREENS

1 THE MIRACLE OF GREENS

We can only appreciate the miracle of a sunrise if we have waited in the darkness. —AUTHOR UNKNOWN

I GET GOOSE BUMPS EVERY TIME I READ ABOUT PHOTOSYNTHESIS. Greens are the only living thing in the world that can transform sunshine into the food that all creatures can consume. There would be no life on our planet without green leaves. The life purpose of all greens is to produce chlorophyll. Dedicated to maximum possible chlorophyll production, green leaves grow, stretch, spread, and quickly take over available space under the sun. That is why we have to constantly cut, clip, and trim the grass, bushes, and trees around us.

Chlorophyll is a miraculous substance, in essence liquefied sunshine. The chlorophyll molecule is the basis for every form of carbohydrate on our planet. That means there is no sugar, honey, potato, spaghetti, rice, or bread that did not originate from a molecule of chlorophyll. All of the energy in food comes from the sun. Plants wisely utilize the sugars created from chlorophyll. As plants don't have their own legs and cannot move, they purposely make their fruit sweet in order to attract animals, insects, birds, and humans to help spread their seeds. That is why fruits look so attractive to us. They are brightly colored, sweet, and smell enticing. Another large part of the sugars made from chlorophyll is transferred to the roots. As you know, the roots of plants have a sweet taste; for example, carrots, beets, yams, potatoes, and turnips. For this reason a large percentage of the world's sugar is produced from root vegetables. All of this leaves one to wonder what the purpose of sweetness in roots could be. Whom can they attract, hidden in the ground, hairy and dirty? There are countless varieties of fungi, microbes, amoebas, bacteria, and microorganisms whose lives depend on the sugar in plant roots. In *Teaming with Microbes,* Jeff Lowenfels and Wayne Lewis give us some idea of how crowded the neighborhood is: "A mere teaspoon of good garden soil, as measured by microbial geneticists, contains a billion invisible bacteria, several yards of equally invisible fungal hyphae, several thousand protozoa, and a few dozen nematodes."[1] These microorganisms all have a big sweet tooth, consuming sugar from the roots of plants and multiplying. They transform organic matter such as dead animals and plants into inorganic minerals. The richness and fertility of the soil is totally dependent on microorganism activity. Without microorganisms, soil turns into dust. The roots of plants are covered with tiny hairs called rhizoids. Through these rhizoids, plants absorb dissolved mineral compounds from the soil when they drink water. As water enters the root hairs and moves through the plant, it carries nutrients to all parts of the plant.

The plant's main purpose for accumulating nutrients is to develop future seeds, which require a high density of nutrients to fulfill their function of reproduction. First, they need to endure a variety of weather conditions such as frost, drought, wind, rain, or heat. In addition to needing strong immunity and the ability to survive any number of circumstances, including the possibility of spending many hours in someone's digestive tract, seeds need to be able to remain dormant for extremely long periods before the proper conditions to sprout arrive. Nutrient density ensures the survival of the seed for hundreds, even thousands of years. In her article on the Svalbard Global Seed Vault in Norway, Martha Hunter Shepard describes seeds' extraordinary potential for survival: "The longest-lasting seed we know of is the sorghum. We have some indication that in certain conditions it could survive some 20,000 years."[2] After the seeds germinate, they still need a lot of energy and nutrition in order to sprout and survive. We see how sprouts of grass sometimes grow

---

[1]Jeff Lowenfels and Wayne Lewis, *Teaming with Microbes* (Portland, OR: Timber Press, 2006).

[2]Martha Hunter Shepard, "Banking on the Future," *Rhodes Magazine* 15 (Fall 2008).

through a thick layer of asphalt, moving rocks or thick layers of clay. The sprouts should be able to survive after heavy animals step on them or nibble at them. If seeds didn't have the necessary nutrition, this wouldn't be possible. This is why plants work hard to feed their underground supply of microorganisms and harvest their minerals.

Plants begin to accumulate nutrients long before their seeds are formed. There is no better place for accumulating and storing nutrients than in the leaves. *This puts greens in the category of the most nutritious foods on the planet.* One may ask, "Aren't seeds the most nutritious part of the plant, then?" While seeds are indeed rich in nutrients, plants don't want their "babies" to be eaten, and therefore protect their seeds by saturating them with all kinds of inhibitors, alkaloids, and other poisonous ingredients.

The best time to harvest greens is before the formation of seeds, because that is when green leaves contain the highest concentration of nutrients. After a plant blossoms, nutrients begin to accumulate inside its seeds. Once the seeds are gone, there are almost no nutrients left in the leaves. They turn yellow and brown, bitter and tough, and eventually fall off the plant so that the remaining nutrients return to the soil and the plant can rest until the next growing season.

In the next chapter we'll look at why harnessing the miraculous nutrition of greens is so crucial for our health.

2 GREENS, THE KEY INGREDIENT IN HUMAN NUTRITION

We know the truth, not only by reason, but also by the heart.
—BLAISE PASCAL

HAVE YOU EVER NOTICED HOW MANY GREEN LEAVES ARE CONSTANTLY growing on this planet? I don't think it is possible to estimate the amount of green mass on the earth. I only know that the prevailing color on our planet is green because of green leaves.

When something is as abundant as greens, we tend to consider it insignificant. Eventually we stop noticing it. For many of us in our busy lives, greens have been reduced to a part of the landscape. Some people view greens as food for the animals. For some folks, greens are a plain nuisance—there are leaves to rake, grass to cut, and weeds to pull. Similarly, we have come to take the greens on our plates for granted.

Yet green leaves are vital for the survival of all living beings on our planet, including humans. In fact, green leaves are as essential for human existence as water, air, and sunlight. I have conducted a lot of research and found that the nutritional composition of greens matches human nutritional needs amazingly well. Greens contain all the essential minerals, vitamins, and even amino acids that humans need for optimal health. The only nutrient not found in greens is vitamin B12. You can find more information about the nutritional value of greens in my book *Green for Life*.[3]

I have found much evidence that green leaves have been a primary staple in the diets of humans from the beginning of time. According to archaeological research, skeletons of the first humans were discov-

---

[3]Victoria Boutenko, *Green for Life* (Ashland, OR: Raw Family Publishing, 2005).

ered in eastern Africa,[4] where the climate at that time was a tropical rain forest. After studying these bones, scientists concluded that humans first lived in the upper canopy level of trees. Examination of their large and square molars, covered with thick enamel, suggests that prehistoric humans ate green leaves along with fruit, blossoms, seeds, bark, and insects.[5]

Documented evidence of the popularity of greens goes back as far as early medieval times. For example, according to German researcher P. Hanelt, "a number of leafy crucifers that no longer exist were used throughout Europe as salad vegetables and scurvy remedies from the sixteenth through the nineteenth centuries."[6] Another scientific researcher tells us how greens "such as cabbage, radish, turnip, mustard, and horseradish flourished throughout Europe by the sixteenth century. Cabbage itself reached cult status as a cure for all diseases."[7]

As my book *12 Steps to Raw Foods* discusses in greater detail, greens have been a staple in the human diet for thousands of years. Throughout human history, people consumed almost exclusively wholesome natural products grown in rich, healthy soil. This way of eating underwent a dramatic shift approximately 180 years ago, when the industrial revolution began. Along with railways, sewing machines, and factories, the processes of canning, refining sugar, and milling white flour were invented. These three innovations were the major contributors to an unprecedented shift in the human diet. While people eagerly embraced convenient, inexpensive, and "progressive" ways of eating, they dramatically reduced their consumption of wholesome foods, especially green vegetables. They replaced highly nutritious natural products with white flour, white sugar,

---

[4]N. Boauz, *Quarry: Closing in on the Missing Link* (New York: The Free Press, 1993).
[5]Victoria Boutenko, *12 Steps to Raw Foods* (Berkeley, CA: North Atlantic Books, 2007).
[6]P. Hanelt, "Lesser-known or Forgotten Cruciferous Vegetables and Their History," *Acta Horticulturae*, no. 459 (1998): 39–45.
[7]G. R. Fenwick, R. K. Heaney, and W. J. Mullin, "Glucosinolates and Their Breakdown Products in Food and Food Plants," *CRC Critical Reviews in Food Science and Nutrition* 18 (1983): 123–201.

hydrogenated oils, artificial additives, and many other heavily processed foods.

Within a matter of years, eating predominantly processed and refined foods became commonplace and, like riding a bicycle and using electricity, was considered a symbol of progress, similar to having a computer and cell phone today. No one suspected that these new foods were high in calories and low in nutrition; on the contrary, most consumers believed that canned, refined, and other processed foods were easier to digest than whole foods. When people began developing various symptoms of deficiencies, they did not associate their illnesses with their newly acquired eating habits. The invention and incorporation of artificial fertilizers, preservatives, and other toxic chemicals further added to nutritional deficiencies. Within several decades, four illnesses spread as a direct result of consuming food depleted of essential nutrients: scurvy, rickets, beriberi, and pellagra. Each of these diseases became epidemic, and thousands of lives were lost. For example, in 1915 more than ten thousand people died of pellagra in the United States alone.[8]

At that time the majority of doctors didn't connect the cause of these diseases with lack of nutrition and therefore they searched for a cure beyond food. During the industrial revolution enormous progress was made in the field of chemistry so physicians began prescribing an ever-increasing variety of medical drugs to help their patients. Unfortunately, doctors were unaware that most medicines administered to patients interfered with the absorption of vital nutrients, causing further nutritional deficiencies. Today a great deal of research is available that explains how medical drugs can create nutritional deficiencies in the human body. For example, iron, one of the most essential minerals for human health, can be obtained from a wide variety of foods, both from animal and vegetable sources. However, despite iron's widespread availability, iron deficiency is the most common nutritional deficiency in the United States, affecting 7.8 million adolescent girls and women of childbearing age, and 700,000 chil-

---

[8]www.hbci.com/~wenonah/new/howfindv.htm

dren aged 1–2 years.[9] In her book *Drug-Induced Nutritional Deficiencies,* Dr. Daphne A. Roe explains that iron absorption has been shown to be depressed by such commonly used medicines as aspirin, antacid, and antibiotics.[10] By adding spinach and other greens rich in iron to our diets, we could eliminate the most common nutritional deficiency and possibly improve our immunity to such a degree that we wouldn't have need of medications.

Nowadays it is a well-known fact that nutritional deficiencies were the original cause of scurvy,[11] beriberi, pellagra, and rickets. For instance, scurvy can be safely and effectively treated by simply adding fresh fruits and vegetables to the sufferer's diet. However, until the end of the nineteenth century, "typical cures for scurvy included purging with salt water, bleeding, eating sulphuric acid or vinegar, and smearing mercury paste onto the open sores."[12] No wonder that "more than two million sailors perished from scurvy" during the two centuries prior to discovery of vitamin C. I wonder if in another two centuries science will discover that some scary diseases of today could be treated by just adding fresh organic produce to our diets.

During the nineteenth century, greater use of chemical medical treatments, increased consumption of processed foods, and more widespread use of toxic substances in everyday life greatly contributed to nutritional deficiencies and toxicity among the general populace. Deficiency and toxicity laid the foundation for the rapid decline in public health. Degenerative diseases began to grow considerably. One of those exploding ailments was cancer.

The oldest known description of human cancer is found in an Egyptian papyrus written between 3000–1500 BC.[13] However, according

---

[9]"Iron deficiency—United States, 1999–2000." *Morbidity and Mortality Weekly Report,* October 11, 2002.

[10]Daphne A. Roe, MD, *Drug-Induced Nutritional Deficiencies* (Westport, CT: AVI Publishing Company, Inc., 1978).

[11]Stephen R. Bown, *Scurvy: How a Surgeon, a Mariner, and a Gentleman Solved the Greatest Medical Mystery of the Age of Sail.* (Markham, Ontario, Canada: Thomas Allen & Son, 2003).

[12]Ibid.

[13]www.cancer.org

to Dr. Max Gerson, cancer continued to be an exceptionally rare disease until the beginning of the industrial revolution.[14] During the nineteenth century the numbers of people diagnosed with cancer started to grow rapidly in developed countries. By 1900, 64 out of every 100,000 Americans died from cancer. These already high numbers continued to grow and tripled by 2000.[15] Now we are told that by 2010 cancer will become the leading cause of death worldwide.[16]

Today, as we continue to increase the amount of processed foods in our diets, the level of public health is falling so quickly that we can observe the dramatic plunge even in the course of one generation. I am only fifty-four, but in my short lifetime I can clearly observe the decline in the health of contemporary youth. For example, when I was in middle school, among the forty students in my class there was only one boy who wore glasses. Nobody wore braces, and there was only one overweight girl, who was made fun of by everyone else. Recently I was teaching a class at a local middle school, and I noticed that a third of the class wore very stylish glasses, many students had braces, many were overweight, and most had acne. On top of that, their teacher told me that several of his students had been diagnosed with attention deficit disorder (ADD) and that numerous children from the class were on different kinds of medications, including antidepressants. Obviously the process of deterioration of our health is continuing, and maybe even escalating.

You and I belong to approximately the seventh generation of people living on predominantly processed food. White flour, white sugar, artificial additives, and many other components of processed foods have contributed to the deficiency and toxicity that modern people have. I consider the dramatic reduction of green vegetables in our diet to be by far the most detrimental choice that we have ever made

---

[14]Max Gerson, MD, *A Cancer Therapy: Results of Fifty Cases and the Cure of Advanced Cancer by Diet Therapy : A Summary of 30 Years of Clinical Experimentation* (Greenfield Center, NY: Greenfield Review Press, 1997).

[15]*U.S. News and World Report,* December 27, 1999.

[16]N. Mulcahy, "Cancer to Become Leading Cause of Death Worldwide by 2010," *Medscape Medical News,* December 10, 2008.

for our health. Here we are in the twenty-first century, with "over 50 percent of Americans deficient in the five most important nutrients and over 80 percent of Americans deficient in one or more essential nutrients," according to the USDA.[17] Our deficiencies continue to accumulate and have already reached such an extent that our skeletal and facial features have begun to change. For example, from lack of calcium, vitamin D, and other essential nutrients, the facial bones of many people are underdeveloped, causing a constriction of the dental arches, which results in tooth crowding. According to Dr. Weston A. Price, "this is a typical expression of inadequate nutrition of the parents."[18] Most young people today have jaws that are so narrow and short that there is simply not enough space for all of their teeth. The majority of our daughters and sons are compelled to remove their wisdom teeth, even when there are no cavities in them. Furthermore, after the painful extraction of all four wisdom teeth, their jaws are often still too narrow for the rest of their teeth. It's common for young people to wear braces so their crowded teeth don't grow crookedly.

Some years ago I read in *Survival in the 21st Century*[19] by Viktoras Kulvinskas that smaller earlobes in humans suggest weak genetic inheritance. I have spent countless hours in libraries looking through archives of photographs taken around the world in the last one hundred and fifty years. My observation is that in the West we are seeing smaller ear lobes with each generation. Vitamin K is crucial for ear cartilage, and for all cartilage elsewhere in the human body. Coincidentally, this vitamin can be found almost exclusively in green leaves. As pregnant mothers and babies typically do not consume enough greens, babies don't have enough vitamin K, and thus with each generation their ears become a little smaller. I speculate that the rest of

---

[17]www.ars.usda.gov/Services/docs.htm?docid=15656

[18]W. A. Price, DDS, *Nutrition and Physical Degeneration* (La Mesa, CA: Price Pottinger Nutrition Foundation, 2003).

[19]Viktoras P. Kulvinskas, *Survival in the 21st Century* (Fairfield, IA: 21st Century Publications, 1981).

our organs that contain cartilage are also affected by a lack of vitamin K. I wonder if the back problems that thirty-one million Americans[20] suffer from, along with more than two hundred thousand knee replacements per year,[21] are also connected to the lack of vitamin K and consistent shortage of greens in our diet. Vibrant health is not possible without the regular consumption of vitamin K.

Vitamin K deficiency has been linked to the following disorders:[22]

skin cancer
liver cancer
heavy menstrual bleeding
nose bleeds
hemorrhaging
easy bruising
osteoporosis
hematomas

Vitamin K deficiency has also been linked to the following birth defects:

shortened fingers
cupped ears
flat nasal bridges
underdevelopment of the nose, mouth, and mid-face
mental retardation
neural tube defects

Unfortunately, according to the USDA 2003 *Annual Performance Report,* "Vitamin K is the least studied vitamin."[23] All green leaves are abundant in this important, overlooked vitamin.

---

[20]A. Kugel, "Carpal Tunnel Syndrome and Chronic Back Pain—A Thing of the Past with Ergonomics," *Medical News Today,* July 9, 2005.

[21]D. Heck, "Revision Rates after Knee Replacement in the United States," *Medical Care* 36, no. 5 (May 1998):661–669.

[22]http://wiki.answers.com/Q/What_does_vitamin_K_deficiency_cause

[23]www.usda.gov

Vitamin K is only one of countless nutrients that are crucial for human health. Today nutritional deficiencies and body toxicity are quickly becoming the norm. By bringing greens back into our everyday menu we can slow down and even reverse the degeneration of our health. Green smoothies are the best way to achieve this goal.

3 THE FIRST GREEN SMOOTHIE

When the solution is simple, God is answering. —ALBERT EINSTEIN

FOR DECADES DIETICIANS HAVE BEEN EDUCATING THE PUBLIC ABOUT the benefits of greens, but it was never clear how best to incorporate fresh greens into everyone's daily diet. The only option for eating greens seemed to be the salad. The problem is that in our industrialized world, the taste of greens is not as appealing as the stimulating taste of processed foods. That is why despite Popeye cartoons and Jolly Green Giant advertisements, mothers pushing broccoli on their children, wheatgrass shots in juice bars, and a variety of green powders becoming available in recent years, greens still remained a nonessential side dish or even an unpleasant requirement for the majority of consumers.

That was also true for me. I knew I needed to eat greens but disliked the taste of them. By 2004 I had already been eating a raw food diet for more than ten years,[24] and although switching to an all-raw diet had allowed me to reverse my most serious conditions—edema, arrhythmia, and depression—I still wasn't experiencing the most vibrant health that I was looking for.

In search of the perfect human diet, I decided to look for an animal genetically close to human beings. I found that chimpanzees share an estimated 99.4 percent of their genes with humans. At the same time, these animals possess an extremely strong natural immunity to AIDS, hepatitis C, cancer, and other fatal human illnesses. I was thinking

---

[24]For a more complete story of the Boutenko family on a raw diet, see Appendix 3.

that if we share 99.4 percent the same genes, our diets should be 99.4 percent similar. It appeared that the opposite was true; that is, the Standard American Diet is about 99 percent different from the diet of wild chimpanzees. See for yourself:

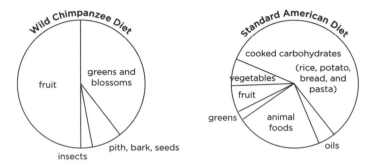

The Standard American Diet is almost 100 percent cooked or processed, while the diet of chimpanzees is 100 percent raw and whole foods. As you can see from the charts below, even the diet of the typical raw foodist resembles the diet of chimpanzees by only 50 percent.

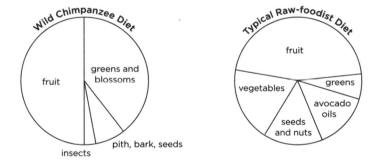

When I recognized how many greens we humans are supposed to consume daily, it became clear to me that I had to come up with an utterly new approach to our diet. From the study of human anatomy I learned that for the best possible absorption, greens have to enter the digestive tract in liquefied form. Greens are high in cellulose, which makes them difficult for the digestive system to break down. In perfectly healthy human bodies without any nutritional deficiencies, greens are liquefied by two processes: first, by thorough chewing, and then by being mixed with stomach acid. Unfortunately, many people today don't have normal levels of hydrochloric acid in their stomach due to mineral deficiencies, particularly of zinc.

You can ask your doctor to perform a stomach acid test on you. How might you know that you have low stomach acid? If you ever vomited as a child, you might remember that the acids from your stomach burned your throat to such an extent that it hurt for several hours. Maybe you can compare this experience with another incident of vomiting later in your life. Do you remember whether or not the burning sensation was still present, weaker, or not felt at all? That might be an indication of a reduced level of hydrochloric acid in your stomach.

People who cannot chew their food thoroughly and who have low hydrochloric acid eventually stop enjoying greens and even develop a distaste for them. This is a defense mechanism of the human body, as if it is telling us, "Honey, you are not able to digest these greens, and they only become a burden on your digestive system, so I'm going to make you nauseous so you stop eating greens completely." It is a vicious cycle: as humans consume more processed food, they become increasingly deficient in nutrients. Then, being unable to create stomach acid, they stop consuming greens and become even more deficient. Their health continues to deteriorate.

When I first began researching the details of digesting greens, I was already missing my most important molars and my stomach acid was extremely low, so I started looking for a way of liquefying large quantities of greens. At first I decided to blend dark leafy greens in a high-speed blender. However, after doing so, when I opened the lid I had to quickly close it as the smell was unbearable. I knew right away that I couldn't possibly drink that mixture, but I knew that I was on the right track. Blender load after blender load was poured into the compost. Several days passed before I came across a paragraph in Jane Goodall's book about chimpanzees in which she mentioned that sometimes chimpanzees would take a piece of fruit, roll it in a green leaf, and eat it as a sandwich. I stared at that paragraph, thinking it was poor food-combining for humans. But then I thought that maybe chimps know better.

So I peeled some bananas and blended them with kale. With trepidation I opened the lid of the blender. To my relief, the smell of bananas masked the smell of chlorophyll. Despite being bright green in color, my smoothie smelled great. I was so excited that I began drinking it right from the blender. I tasted my supergreen drink and discovered that the bananas also dominated the taste of chlorophyll. I was stunned by this discovery. I was able to trick my body into consuming a large amount of greens without any resistance. I didn't feel nauseous. In fact, I ecstatically enjoyed greens for the first time in my life. This discovery marked the beginning of my own green smoothie revolution.

As I was drinking my very first green smoothie, it dawned on me that my children could also enjoy eating greens this way. And my friends, neighbors, coworkers, students, and, oh, my goodness, the whole world too! At this point I started dancing in my office, and then in the street. I made more green smoothies, took a stack of paper cups, and went outside. I offered smoothies to my neighbors and to passers-by. I wanted to see if they would also like the taste of green smoothies, and they did. I couldn't stop laughing and shouting with delight. I recognized that green smoothies were a perfect solution for people like me, of whom there were millions.

4 THE IMPORTANCE OF ROTATING GREENS IN YOUR SMOOTHIES

To improve is to change; to be perfect is to change often.
—WINSTON CHURCHILL

WHEN I FIRST CAME UP WITH THE GREEN SMOOTHIE IDEA, I DECIDED I needed the darkest possible green leaves in my smoothies so that I could undo the damage of not consuming enough greens earlier in my life. That is why for several months I was almost exclusively blending dinosaur kale. This green received its name because it resembles the skin of a dinosaur. Also known as Italian kale, it belongs to the *Brassica* family and is found in most supermarkets around the world. Valya and I especially enjoyed smoothies made with this kale. However, after three months of drinking the same recipe, we started to notice a feeling of slight numbness on our faces. I immediately connected this symptom with the green smoothie, as it was the only change in our family's lifestyle. I remember thinking, *Oh, no! I don't want to give up our beloved smoothies.* I started to research the nutritional content of greens and soon discovered that there was a reason for our symptoms.

Green leaves are typically the most nutritious part of a plant, and creatures naturally want to eat them. Plants carry a trace of alkaloids in their leaves to ensure that animals will move on to eat other green plants and will not exterminate any one species. Although alkaloids are poisonous in large quantities, in small quantities they cannot hurt you, and even strengthen the immune system. The science of homeopathy is based on this principle. However, if you keep consuming kale, or spinach, or any other single green for many weeks without rotation, eventually the same type of alkaloids can accumulate in your body and cause unwanted symptoms of poisoning. Most greens contain different kinds of alkaloids, which is why, by rotating the variety of greens in our smoothies, we can avoid poisoning and strengthen our immunity.

We do not have to rotate our fruits very often because fruits rarely contain alkaloids. In fact, fruits were intended by nature to be eaten in order to spread their seeds. That is why ripe fruit is sweet, aromatic, and bright in color.

You can rotate your greens in any way that is convenient to you. Some people put a different type of green in their smoothie every day. Others put a variety of greens in each smoothie. I recommend rotating a minimum of seven varieties of greens, one for each day of the week. Try to get as much variety as possible. The larger the assortment of greens you consume, the broader the spectrum of vital nutrients your body receives.

While I don't know the exact number of edible greens on our planet, I do know that there are thousands. In his book *Native American Ethnobotany,*[25] Daniel Moerman has listed 1,649 species of edible plants used by Native Americans alone. Since dramatically reducing our consumption of greens in the last two centuries, we have lost our knowledge of most edible greens. Now we have to rely on various people around the world to restore our ability to recognize edible plants. As I travel and meet smoothie drinkers, I collect bits and pieces of information about edible greens. My son Sergei has a hiking company, Harmony Hikes, that takes groups of people out into the wilderness and teaches them to identify edible and poisonous plants. During the spring and summer he shows up with a basket of many different species of plants that we gratefully throw in the blender. Sergei is a big enthusiast of wild edibles and believes that they are nature's true superfoods. He created several short videos about the most common wild edible plants and has placed them on YouTube for your education and enjoyment.

---

[25]Daniel Moerman, *Native American Ethnobotany* (Portland, OR: Timber Press, 1998).

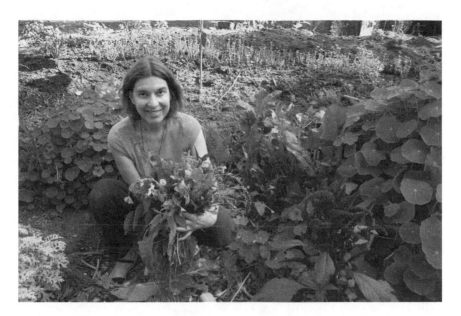

The following is a list of edible greens that can be found in most regions. I would like to acknowledge the biggest contributor to my list, Gabrielle Chavez, an author, teacher, and gardener from Portland, Oregon.

CULTIVATED GREENS

amaranth
arugula (rocket)
bamboo leaves
beet greens
bok choy
cactus, nopal leaves
carrot tops
celery
chard (all types)
collard greens
cucumber leaves
endive
escarole
frisée lettuce
goji (wolfberry) leaves
grape leaves

kale (all types)
mâche
mitsuna
mustard greens
lettuce
   (all types, red and green)
orach
pumpkin or squash leaves
radicchio
radish tops
romaine lettuce
salad burnet
spinach
turnip greens
wheatgrass

WILD EDIBLES AND WEEDS

chickweed

clover

dandelion (greens and flowers)

knotweed

lambsquarters

lovage

malva

miner's lettuce

oxeye daisy flowers and leaves

plantain

purslane

rose leaves and flowers

sorrel

stinging nettles

watercress

wild mustard

wild radish

wild strawberries

wild violets

yellow dock

HERBS

baby dill

basil

bergamot

cilantro

fennel

lemon balm

mint

parsley (Italian or
flat leaf, and curly)

peppermint leaves

shiso

spearmint

stevia

SPROUTS

For variety, we include several kinds of sprouts in our diet, but never more than a handful, and only one or two times per week. From approximately the third to the sixth day of their lives, sprouts contain higher levels of alkaloids as a means of protection against animals nipping them off and killing them.[26] That doesn't mean that sprouts are necessarily dangerous, only that we need to limit our intake. Most sprouts are rich in B vitamins and contain many times more nutrients than the leaves of a fully developed plant because sprouts need more nutrition for their fast growing period. In my green smoothies I use only sprouts that have green leaves on them.

---

[26]Elizabeth Baker, *Unbelievably Easy Sprouting* (Poulsbo, WA: Drelwood, 2000).

alfalfa
broccoli
buckwheat "lettuce" (sprouts)
clover
fenugreek
radish
sunflower

MEDICINAL HERBS

Medicinal herbs are edible but contain higher-than-usual levels of alkaloids and have to be used in smaller amounts. I enjoy a variety of medicinal herbs in my smoothies in the summer, but I always put them in my smoothie with other greens, and not very often. Use them sparingly, and if you're not sure, leave them out.

aloe leaf
borage leaves and flowers
calendula flowers and leaves
cardoon leaves
chervil
cleaver (bedstraw)
clover
comfrey flowers and leaves
fig leaves
filaree
ginkgo
hollyhock flowers
    and leaves
horsetail
Hosta
Japanese maple
    young leaves
Lamium weed
Lapsana communis
    (nipplewort)
Lavatera flowers and leaves
milk thistle
oca
Douglas fir young needles
salsify
sweet cicely

POISONOUS PLANTS

I urge you to exercise caution. There are approximately one hundred and fifty poisonous plants in North America. Be aware and learn to identify the following twenty-two most toxic plants.[27]

---

[27]T. S. Elias and P. A. Dykeman, *Edible Wild Plants: A North American Field Guide* (New York: Sterling, 1990).

American yew	jimsonweed
Atamasco lily	mayapple
baneberry	Ohio buckeye
blue flag	poison hemlock
buttercup	poison ivy
butterfly weed	poison oak
death camas	pokeweed
dogbane	southwestern coral bean
false hellebore	star of Bethlehem
foxglove	water hemlock
horse nettle	yellow flag

List does not include poisonous mushrooms.

Wild edibles always contain more vitamins and minerals than commercially marketed plants. Weeds have not been "spoiled" with farmers' care, in contrast to the "good" plants of the garden. In order to survive in spite of constant weeding, pulling, and spraying, weeds have had to develop strong survival properties. For example, to stay alive without being watered, most weeds have developed unbelievably long roots. Alfalfa's roots grow up to twenty feet long, reaching for the most fertile layers of the soil. As a result, all wild plants possess more nutrients than commercially grown plants. I feel so silly now when I remember how I used to always pull out the "nasty" lambs-quarters from my garden to let my "precious" iceberg lettuce grow. Now I collect seeds of dandelions, stinging nettles, lambsquarters, and other weeds in the fall and grow them in my garden along with kale and spinach to increase the variety of greens in my smoothies.

I enjoy the rich flavor and slightly bitter taste of weeds. In my family we have found that the longer we consume green smoothies, the more we appreciate bitter greens such as dandelion, parsley, endive, escarole, and frisée. During our recent trip to Australia, Valya and I noticed how bitter the greens tasted there. Even chard, spinach, and lettuce, which we consider mild-tasting in the United States, were so bitter there that we wondered if they were different plants. Australian farmers explained to us that their greens grow in volcanic soil, which is very fertile and rich in minerals. I wanted to know if the bitterness of these greens meant they were high in nutrients. I browsed the Internet and found scientific research confirming this to be true. According to University of Washington researcher Adam Drewnowski, "The phytochemicals are antioxidants, and they are all bitter. Antioxidants are chemicals that prevent damage to cells in the body. Avoiding fruits and vegetables that produce bitter sensations in your mouth could translate into a loss of important health benefits. The same chemicals in plants that make for a bitter taste may also prevent cancer and heart disease."[28] Even knowing about the wonderful benefits of bitter greens, many people would still not be able to consume a lot them due to their unpleasant taste. Blending with fruit turns bitter greens into an enjoyable treat. By including bitter greens in your smoothies you might acquire a taste for them. When I started drinking green smoothies five years ago, I couldn't tolerate the bitter taste of dandelions and blended them together with a lot of sweet fruit. Now dandelions have become one of my favorite salad greens.

Once in a while I read in the news or receive an e-mail about kale, spinach, parsley, or some other green having a toxic ingredient and therefore being dangerous for human consumption. This may be true, but not to such a degree that we should exclude any particular green from our diet. Let us learn to increase the variety of greens in our diet and to constantly rotate them for better nutritional results.

---

[28] Adam Drewnowski, PhD, and Carmen Gomez-Carneros, "Bitter Bounty: Worst-Tasting Produce May Be the Best for You," *American Journal of Clinical Nutrition*, December 2000.

5 BLENDING VERSUS JUICING

To manage a system effectively, you might focus on the interactions of the parts rather than their behavior taken separately.   —PAUL ERLICH

AFTER I PUBLISHED MY FIRST BOOK ABOUT GREEN SMOOTHIES, I received many inquiries from my readers asking whether blending was preferable to juicing. I also heard that some nutritionists were concerned that blending might accelerate the oxidation of food. I was very curious to find the answer for myself and began to research this question.

I decided to conduct a simple experiment. I chose potatoes for my experiment because it is easy to observe the process of oxidation in potatoes. You probably remember an instance when you left a slice of raw potato on your cutting board and observed it turning brown within several minutes. That is why my grandmother used to put peeled potatoes in water, to prevent browning or oxidation.

First I peeled two potatoes so that the color of their peel wouldn't interfere with the results of my experiment. I then juiced one potato in a twin-gear juicer, and blended the other one in a Vita-Mix blender with one cup of water. I placed both cups of fluid on the table and took a photograph of them. I took photographs frequently for two days. The potato juice started to turn brown within a matter of minutes and became dark brown by the end of the first hour. The blended potato stayed almost white for two days. The top of both liquids, which was exposed to the air, turned dark almost instantly. I repeated this experiment three times with different kinds of potatoes and various shapes of glasses. The results were the same.

It was clear that the juiced potato oxidized faster than the blended potato. Since I am not a professional scientist, I decided to seek the

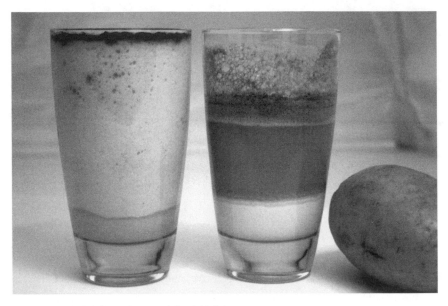

Potato blended (left) and potato juiced (right).

opinion of someone with the appropriate expertise. I went to the local university and consulted with Gregory T. Miller, professor of chemistry at Southern Oregon University. After researching this matter, he wrote the following:

> Browning is the result of oxidation of specific biomolecules in the fruit or vegetable. My students study this in lab, so I have some familiarity with the process (albeit they are studying the enzymatically regulated oxidation). My wife is a winemaker and deals with oxidation of her juice and wine on a regular basis. I also possess a huge number of resources on the oxidation topic in the form of biochemistry, medical, and nutritional books. Here are my thoughts:
>
> Many people believe that the blending process will cause increased oxidation due to thousands of tiny air bubbles getting mixed into the blended liquid. This effectively increases the surface area of oxygen in the liquid and facilitates the oxidation process. However, in grapes at least, I have observed the opposite to be true. The blended grape stays a truer color much longer than when juiced. I believe this observation in grapes to be a result of numerous antioxidants released as the grape is

blended, which breaks open more cells than in juicing. I believe this is what you are seeing with the potato as well.

Potatoes contain numerous antioxidants. This may come as a surprise to many people because of the pale color of many varietals. Among others, potatoes are rich sources of phenolics, flavonoids, carotenoids, and anthocyanins. The concentration of each varies with the type of potato. Since your potatoes are skinless (where the greatest concentration of the tyrosinase enzyme is located), I believe the blending process releases a much higher percentage of these antioxidants from the tissue than the juicing process.

It is also possible that, in many fruits and vegetables, the bulk of the fiber released during blending reduces the oxygen saturation in the solution but, if true, I think this is a secondary issue.

I think this experiment explains why it is commonly advised to drink freshly squeezed juice within minutes of making it, and why smoothies can stay fresh for two or three days in the fridge.

In hopes of gathering more scientific feedback, I e-mailed the description of my potato experiment to the twenty-five thousand people on my mailing list. I have received many valuable responses, one of which I found especially helpful and would like to share with you. Michael Donaldson, PhD, a chemical engineering graduate from Cornell University, recreated the potato experiment. His conclusions were as follows:

- The initial oxidation in the blender and in juicing was of equal speed.
- By the next morning, the juice had more color, while the blend did not. The blended liquid was much thicker, so the color formed on the top did not migrate down into the solution like it did with the juice.
- I disagree with those who say that blending is very destructive, or much more so than juicing.

I appreciate this feedback from scientists and hope there will be more research done soon on this important subject. So far, my conclusion is that there are benefits both to blending and juicing.

The main advantage of juice over smoothies is that juice requires little digesting and can be assimilated immediately into the bloodstream, allowing the digestive system to rest. This quality of juice is particularly important for people who suffer from severe nutritional deficiencies or have a highly irritable digestive system. People with these conditions often cannot tolerate any fiber at all, and juice can provide invaluable nourishment for them. Green juice has been shown to be extremely beneficial for people suffering from cancer and other degenerative diseases.[29]

However, I agree with Dr. Doug Graham that juices are a "fractured food," missing the essential component of fiber along with its antioxidants. When we consume enough fiber, we take a load off of our bodies by improving our elimination. Toxins often build up in the colon, and fiber cleans them out. When most toxins have been removed by fiber, the body has a greater ability to absorb nutrients, thus improving digestion. Humans could not live on juices alone, whereas green smoothies are a complete food.

If I don't have a blender around me, I juice. One time, I gave my blender to my brother because I thought that he needed it more than I. While waiting for my new Vita-Mix, I was juicing greens because I could not live without them. But I quickly got tired of the limited variety of flavors and noticed that I felt hungrier and had to add more salads to my menu since the juices were not as filling as smoothies. In contrast, smoothies are very filling; I can live on them for days, even weeks. I know of people who have chosen to live on smoothies for several weeks or months with beneficial results. You will find the extraordinary story of Clent Manich's green smoothie experiment in Appendix 1 and 2.

For everyday use and for the majority of people, I believe green smoothies to be optimal. They are fast to make, delicious, and nutritious at the same time. No other food can compete with the two main advantages of green smoothies: nutritional value and practicality.

---

[29]Max Gerson, MD, *A Cancer Therapy: Results of Fifty Cases and the Cure of Advanced Cancer by Diet Therapy: A Summary of 30 Years of Clinical Experimentation* (Greenfield Review Press, Greenfield Center, NY, 1997).

6 A GREEN SMOOTHIE Q&A

THROUGH MY WORKSHOPS, LECTURES, AND WEB SITE, I AM ALWAYS fielding questions about green smoothies. In fact, this book was written in part to address questions that have come up since the publication of my previous book, *Green for Life*. Answers to many of those questions have been incorporated in other chapters. These are some of the other issues most frequently asked about.

Question: How many greens should I eat every day?

Victoria: There is a big difference between consuming greens as a salad or in blended form. Our bodies can assimilate several times more vital nutrients from blended greens than from chewed greens because the blender breaks down food into much smaller particles. Some high-speed blenders can even break open plant cell walls. In comparison, salads require thorough chewing, and we don't generally chew sufficiently to derive the full benefits from what we eat. Salads are also served with oils and other spices, which significantly slow down digestion. If you prefer to eat greens as a salad, I estimate that you should consume at least two bunches of greens (or six packed cups) per day. If you drink your greens in blended form, then one bunch (three packed cups) per day will be sufficient.

Question: Where can I get my protein?

Victoria: This is the most popular question asked in my lectures. I believe that we inherited the fear of not having enough protein in our diet from the beginning of the last century. In his 520-page book on fundamental nutritional research published in 1922, Dr. McCollum stated: "Through studies it became established that the body of an animal or the tissues of a plant consist essentially of proteins, carbohydrates, fats, and a series of related substances. Several other prominent components ... are not essential."[30] Later in the same book he concluded, "Protein is the most prominent organic component of the body." Perhaps this straightforward conclusion coming from a professor of Chemical Hygiene and Public Health at the Johns Hopkins University in Baltimore seemed so conclusive that we believe it to this day. Since then nutrition scientists have discovered hundreds of different nutrients that are crucially important for human health. For instance, some researchers estimate that there are up to forty thousand phytonutrients, which we have barely begun to study. I often wonder why nobody is asking, "Where can I get my phytonutrients?" By the way, we can get most of them, along with protein, from fresh greens. Consider this: cow's milk was green grass just four hours before the cow was milked. For more information about protein in greens please see my book *Green for Life,* where I devote a full chapter to the subject. When researching this topic I discovered a great deal of fascinating but little-known information, for example, that one pound of kale contains even more protein than the daily allowance recommended by the USDA.

Question: Can we use wheatgrass in our smoothies?

Victoria: Wheatgrass adds beautifully to the variety of green smoothies. Sometimes I purchase a small pot of wheatgrass in soil, the kind often sold for pets. Wheatgrass grows very fast, and I usually get three harvests of grass clippings from a small pot for my green smoothies. However, please remember that wheatgrass, like any green, contains a minute amount of alkaloids and should be rotated.

---

[30]E. V. McCollum, PhD, ScD, *The Newer Knowledge of Nutrition* (New York: The Macmillan Company, 1922).

Question: I make my green smoothies with a lot of sweet fruit and even dates, raisins, figs, and prunes. I'm worried that I consume too many sweets. Should I use less?

Victoria: You can put more sweet fruit and even dates in the smoothie for a beginner or for a child. Most people are not yet accustomed to the taste of chlorophyll and simply will not drink it if it tastes too "green" to them. I think it is very important to prepare smoothies that are so delicious that everyone will look forward to them. Based on my observation and feedback from other smoothie drinkers, most people naturally start to crave greener smoothies in several weeks. On the other hand, some people who were trying to be too perfect too quickly prepared "supergreen" smoothies from the very beginning. They complained that the green smoothies tasted awful, and they quit, never wanting to try them again. If you are sensitive to sugar for such reasons as diabetes, candida, or hypoglycemia, you may have to start with less sweet smoothies by adding low–glycemic index fruit such as berries and apples. As another option, you can prepare savory smoothies made from greens and nonstarchy vegetables such as tomatoes, cucumbers, celery, bell peppers, and others.

Question: How many smoothies should I drink per day?

Victoria: You can enjoy as many green smoothies as you like. Sometimes I drink only one quart, but more often I drink two, three, and even four quarts a day.

Question: Can I freeze greens if I cannot use them all at once?

Victoria: I have never frozen my greens, but if I lived in a northern country and had, for example, a large harvest of spinach, I would freeze it and use it over time. Frozen greens will still be more nutritious than cooked greens. However, if you have access to fresh greens, they are significantly more nutritious and tastier than frozen.

Question: How long do smoothies keep?

Victoria: Green smoothies are best when fresh, but if necessary they can be kept up to three days. When I am home I make fresh smoothies every morning, but when I travel I make two to three gallons of smoothies ahead of time and keep them in a cooler in my car. I drink my green smoothies as long as they are fresh. I am surprised that often after three days they still taste good and have a brilliant green color.

Question: Do you think it is better to use powdered greens in green smoothies as opposed to fresh greens?

Victoria: If we rotate our greens and consume at least one quart of green smoothie per day, we receive an optimal amount of nutrients. I recommend leaving green powders for the times when fresh greens are not accessible, for example while traveling. I do not think that dried greens are nearly as vibrant or nutritious as fresh greens. My daughter Valya recently decided to further explore the theory of dried versus fresh greens at a friend's horse farm. Valya preformed an experiment by offering six horses the option of eating fresh grass or high-quality dried hay. Six out of six horses chose the fresh greens over the dry hay.

Question: Should I avoid eating spinach because it has oxalic acid?

Victoria: The oxalic acid in food is considered harmful because it can combine with calcium and may leach the body of this important mineral. For some reason, everyone knows about the oxalic acid in spinach, but they are not aware of the oxalic acid content in many other commonly eaten foods such as grains, beans, and especially coffee and tea. While spinach is loaded with calcium, which minimizes the loss of this mineral from your body, coffee has none. I would be more concerned about the oxalic acid content in coffee and other products than in spinach. At the same time, even though the oxalic acid content in spinach is minute, if you do not rotate your greens and use only spinach for many weeks, you may accumulate oxalic acid and experience symptoms of poisoning. Remember, rotate your greens!

Question: What about vitamin B12, which vegans don't receive from plants?

Victoria: Vitamin B12 is the only nutrient that we cannot get from plants. There is a lot of research currently going on regarding B12. The USDA recommends getting this vitamin from animal products via meat, eggs, or dairy products. Many vegans and raw foodists take vitamin B12 supplements. Dr. Vivian Vetrano and other doctors of natural hygiene state that vitamin B12 is made by bacteria in the intestinal tract if it is healthy. In my family we have not had symptoms of B12 deficiency even though we have never taken supplements of this vitamin. So as you can see, there is some conflicting information about this important issue. Scientific research has shown that vitamin B12 deficiency is dangerous for human health, so take supplements if you have to.

Question: How can I identify the weeds that I can eat?

Victoria: We have to be cautious when picking wild edibles because there are poisonous plants in nature. Go to the library or visit your local bookstore and find a book that pertains to your local area. I live in southern Oregon, and some of our weeds here are different from those of other regions. I recommend that you first learn about several well-known weeds that are common throughout the United States and other parts of the world. Some examples of wild edibles include plantain, dandelion, chickweed, miner's lettuce, and stinging nettle. These weeds are high in nutrition, and you can easily find them locally.

There are many helpful books available about wild edibles written for different regions. The Internet is a great resource for identifying wild greens and weeds. For example, you may want to collect plantain (a wild edible, unrelated to the banana plant) because it is high in protein and vitamins A and D, and it lowers cholesterol and blood pressure. If you go to Yahoo or Google and search the name of the plant under the "image" tabs, you will find several images of plantain displayed, enough to identify this wild green.

Question: Is it beneficial to add any fat to smoothies?

Victoria: I do not recommend adding fat to your green smoothie. I believe that the formula of the green smoothie—fruit, greens, and water—is perfect and needs no improvement. Any additional ingredients will take away from the nutritional value of the green smoothie. However, I understand that each person is unique and may have different needs. You can add anything you want to your smoothies. What is most important is that you keep drinking them regularly.

Question: Since I started drinking green smoothies, my stool has become green. Is this normal?

Victoria: When the level of stomach acid is low, one may find pieces of undigested food in the stool, and its color may reflect the color of the food consumed, such as red from beets or green from green smoothies. After daily consumption of green smoothies, the body receives plenty of nourishment, and the level of stomach acid begins to normalize. Eventually you will always have the same color stool despite your food intake. Normal stool should be light brown in color, odorless, well formed, and not stick to the toilet. It leaves the body easily without straining or discomfort.

Question: I started eating a raw food diet and drinking green smoothies three days ago, and I feel constipated. What did I do wrong?

Victoria: When people eat predominately refined food, which is low in fiber, their bowels become sluggish. For this reason, the contents of the large intestines are moved not from peristalsis but rather from being pushed by the following meals. Raw food is high in fiber and nutrition, and it consists of about 90 percent water. That is a big change for the intestines to get used to. It may take a couple of weeks, and sometimes longer, for the intestines to heal, for their muscle tone to improve, and for them to start working properly.

7 GREEN SMOOTHIES FOR OUR CHILDREN

Children are the world's most valuable resource and its best hope for the future. —JOHN F. KENNEDY

WHEN I LEARNED FROM MY OLDEST SON STEPHAN THAT HIS WIFE, Tasia, was expecting a child, I immediately purchased and sent them a Vita-Mix blender. Knowing that Stephan and Tasia did not eat a raw food diet, I asked them to make only one simple change: to add at least one cup of green smoothie to their daily diet. I explained that this simple addition would provide important nourishment not only for the baby but also for the parents, and it would help them to be vibrant and balanced in time for the baby's arrival. They promised to follow my instructions since they were both excited and happy to do everything possible to have a healthy baby. At first they didn't like the taste of the greens in the smoothie and had to double the amount of fruit, which made the smoothie more of a yellow color rather than green. However, within weeks they reported that they were starting to enjoy more greens both in their smoothie and in their salads.

A couple of months later, Tasia excitedly shared with me that she felt the baby kicking more vigorously after she had a green smoothie. Her doctor told her that this was a great sign. She tried not to miss even one day of smoothie drinking. Every morning upon waking, she blended enough smoothie for herself and for Stephan to take to work in a thermos. Tasia admitted that she was looking forward to the end of the pregnancy so that she could have a break from this routine. Little did she know....

My first darling grandchild, Nic, was born on December 1, 2004. Within days of his birth, Nic's parents learned that he wouldn't sleep through the night if Tasia didn't drink her smoothie that day. Moreover, he would be cranky and moody without his habitual portion of nutrition. The blending continued.

Nic was fed his first teaspoon of green smoothie when he turned six months old. He loved it right away. He quickly made the connection between the roaring sound of the Vita-Mix and his favorite drink. Every time he heard the familiar noise, he would get excited and laugh. As soon as Nic learned how to crawl, he would crawl into the kitchen and bang on the fridge, yelling *"vvv-vvv-vvv,"* demanding a green smoothie. When he learned to walk, he would walk over to the counter where the blender was kept, point a tiny finger, and say *"moo-ee, moo-ee!"* Tasia no longer expects a break from smoothie making any time soon! At the same time, she was happy to learn from Nic's doctor that their child was the healthiest in the entire district, and he requested to see Nic less often than the other children. Green smoothies have become an important addition to Nic's otherwise standard diet.

The majority of children love green smoothies. I recommend that you prepare especially delicious green smoothies for your children and for beginners of any age. I usually make the smoothie for children sweeter than for myself and decorate it nicely with fresh berries. Don't force your children to drink green smoothies. Instead, let them see how much you enjoy this delicious, healthy drink.

For those who already have a child who has built up resistance to greens, we recommend what we call "a shot in the dark." Serve the green smoothie in a cup that is not clear, and have them try it while their attention is focused on something else. If they try this delicious, sweet concoction without paying attention to the green color, they might fall in love with it. I have found that children often love green smoothies even more than adults do. While we offer special recipes for children in this book, kids only need these sweet and mild-tasting smoothies in the very beginning because they will quickly develop a taste for supergreen drinks. Green smoothies are so fast and easy to make that educators and parents are increasingly interested in adopting smoothies into children's diets.

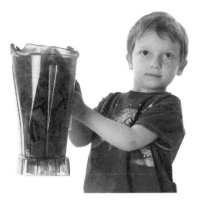

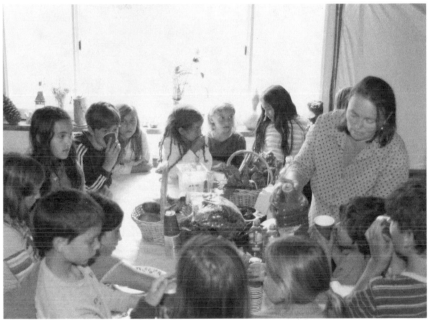

Left: Nic at age three and a half.

Below: Victoria makes smoothies for an eager young audience.

My family and I have visited many schools and demonstrated green smoothie preparation to children and teachers. Usually, after tasting the smoothie and hearing about its benefits, children are willing to try making their own drinks. A word of caution for parents: when you teach your children to eat healthfully, be prepared for them surprise you with a "special treat" such as a shot of wheatgrass juice on your birthday!

8 GREEN SMOOTHIES FOR OUR PETS

We can judge the heart of a man by his treatment of animals.
—IMMANUEL KANT

IN THE WILDERNESS, ALL ANIMALS CONSUME GREEN FOODS REGULARLY. Even polar bears are known to graze on grasses, kelp, and crowberries. All wild animals are notably healthier than household pets. I believe one of the key factors contributing to the poor health of our pets is that in captivity their access to green foods is extremely limited, if not totally absent.

Several years ago, my son Sergei was visiting his friends Jack and Amanda, who had a diabetic cat. This cat had been given insulin shots regularly for many years. When Sergei arrived, his friends were hovering around their cat looking concerned. It appeared their kitty was behaving strangely. It was breathing rapidly and sometimes fainting. Jack ran to the cabinet only to find that they were out of insulin shots. It was a holiday, and all the stores in town were closed. Amanda began to cry, thinking that their beloved pet was about to die. Sergei suggested that they let the cat outside, in case it intuitively knew what might help. Amanda protested, "But he's an indoor cat, and he will get hit by a car if he is let out. He has never been outside in his life!" Sergei replied, "Well, I don't think you have much to lose at this point." They decided to let the cat out, and opened the door. The kitty quickly ran out and went directly to the lawn. He began to vigorously eat grass. All three humans watched the "sick" cat in amazement. Within minutes the kitty was visibly better. He quietly went back in the house and fell asleep on the couch.

Several weeks later, Amanda called Sergei and told him that when they took their cat to the vet, the doctor explained that the cat was misdiagnosed and insisted it never had diabetes to begin with. He said that the cat suffered not from an illness but from malnutrition. Since then, Amanda and Jack have been letting their kitty out and even buying him wheatgrass. The cat acts more playful and looks much healthier than before.

My brother's family lives on a very tight budget and can only afford to buy the cheapest food for their cat, Timothy. Unfortunately, my brother's wife loved houseplants and had a plethora of them all over the apartment. Following his instincts, Timothy consumed one houseplant after another until he had eaten them all up, even the cactuses. I thought they were exaggerating these stories until I had the chance to host Timothy for a weekend while my brother moved. These two days were plenty of time for Timothy to devour my daughter's ferns, palms, and especially aloe vera plants.

Once, while defending her territory, my cat, Masya, got into a brutal fight and had her eye slashed. The veterinarian prescribed scores of antibiotics and other drugs, without which he assured me Masya would lose her eye. Instead of taking his advice, I began giving my cat wheatgrass juice and green smoothies every hour. Her recovery was spectacularly fast and effective. Masya loves greens. If I am working on a salad and happen to drop a leaf of lettuce, she is happy to "vacuum" it up for me. I hear from friends that their dogs instantly fall in love with green smoothies and have no problem consuming them in addition to their regular food.

Greens are healthy for cats and dogs; greens make their fur shine, boost their immune system, prolong life, and protect against cancer. Dogs can safely eat the same green smoothies that you prepare for yourself. For cats you have to prepare a special blend without fruit, as most cats don't like fruit and don't digest it as well.

If your pets don't like green smoothies yet, you may want to teach them. For example, my cat didn't like green smoothies at first, so Valya used an eye dropper to put a few drops in Masya's mouth every time we made one for ourselves. Within a week she was happily licking green smoothie from Valya's palm. Now she enjoys a little bit of

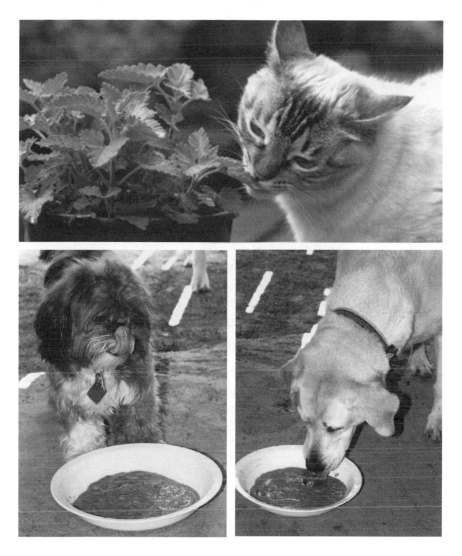

green smoothie a couple of times a week. Our cat's regular serving is two to three tablespoons twice a week.

Our neighbor has two dogs, and they will drink any green smoothie that I offer them; they even got their owner, Nancy, curious about green smoothies. She read *Green for Life* and now enjoys smoothies too! We included a few recipes for your cats and dogs in the recipe section of this book. (Please adjust the quantity of green smoothies for the size of your dog—chihuahuas and labradors will have very different needs!)

Since I live on a mountain slope close to the forest, I decided to check if wild animals would be interested in green smoothes. One evening, I made a gallon of green smoothie out of apples and kale. I poured it in a large bowl and set it outside across from the window. As the sky began to darken, a raccoon came by to have a sip. He was followed by a family of skunks, and even a big deer. Later that night I awoke to a tremendous racket. A huge brown bear had come down to find out if there was any smoothie left over. I was so amazed that I pulled out my video camera and filmed him, but the video turned out too dark. Even though I wouldn't recommend that you conduct such an experiment in your neighborhood, I was astonished with the results. It seems all animals instinctively know they need greens to stay healthy, only they are much more eager to consume them than we are.

9 FOOD COMBINING IN GREEN SMOOTHIES

No law or ordinance is mightier than understanding. —PLATO

THE MOST FREQUENT QUESTION I RECEIVE ABOUT GREEN SMOOTHIES concerns food combining. People ask if it is proper to combine fruits and vegetables in a smoothie. I usually reply that I never combine fruits and vegetables in my smoothies, only fruits and greens. I believe that greens were erroneously placed in the category of vegetables. Greens do not contain starch, and most vegetables do. Both cheese and beef come from a cow, but they belong to different food categories. Similarly, there is a substantial difference between green leaves and vegetables, even though they are often harvested from the same plant. I define "greens" as the flat leaves of a plant, attached to the stem, that can be wrapped around a finger (with a very few exceptions, including nopal cactus leaves and celery). Keeping greens in the same category as vegetables is misleading and can even be harmful to public health. I suggest that our produce departments have at least the following three separate sections: fruits, vegetables, and greens.

And of course, there are many different fruits that are green in color simply because they are unripe. These do not belong in the category of greens. I have received e-mails from readers who started buying unripe, green fruit instead ripe fruit in the mistaken belief that they would be consuming more greens. Most of us know that green bananas are unripe, but don't realize that green grapes, melons, limes, pears, olives, and most green apples and tomatoes are actually unripe yellow fruits. Similarly, green bell peppers are unripe bell peppers. Unripe fruit usually contains enzyme inhibitors, which slow the action of our digestive enzymes and may cause irritation of the intestines. In addition, unripe fruit has a higher starch content and less fruit sugar, which makes it harder to digest. For this reason, I never buy unripe fruit.

I see several benefits in adding greens to other foods. For example, besides having high nutritional value, greens contain a lot of fiber. The fiber in greens slows down the absorption of sugar from fruit. This quality makes drinking green smoothies possible even for people with high sensitivity to sugar, such as those who have diabetes, candida, or hypoglycemia.

In his book *Food Combining Made Easy*,[31] Dr. Herbert Shelton explains that starchy foods have to be eaten alone because starches are digested with enzymes different from those used for any other food group. Combining starchy foods with fruit may cause fermentation and gas. Dr. Shelton has found that combining green vegetables with every food group produces favorable results. Dr. Anne Wigmore, who pioneered raw food in the United States, also taught in her lectures that green leaves are the only food that can be combined with every other food group without any negative effects.

Vegetables such as carrots, beets, broccoli, zucchini, daikon radish, cauliflower, cabbage, Brussels sprouts, eggplant, pumpkin, squash, okra, peas, corn, green beans, and others do not combine well with fruit due to their high starch content. While these vegetables are nutritious and beneficial for our health, their high starch content makes them unsuitable for use in smoothies.

If you do not want to mix sweet fruit into your green smoothies, you can use nonstarchy vegetables or fruit such as tomatoes, cucumbers, bell peppers, avocados, and celery. You can also consider using low–glycemic index fruit such as berries (any kind), apples, cherries, plums, and grapefruit.

So, can we combine greens and fruits in our smoothies? Absolutely.

---

[31]Herbert Shelton, *Food Combining Made Easy* (San Antonio, TX: Dr. Shelton's Health School, 1951).

10 GUIDELINES FOR OPTIMAL GREEN SMOOTHIE CONSUMPTION

Why do I ask for directions? Because I hate wasting time. —HARRISON FORD

TO HELP YOU RECEIVE THE MOST BENEFITS FROM DRINKING GREEN smoothies and to avoid some typical mistakes, I have created the following guidelines:

Prepare your green smoothie first thing in the morning in the amount that you usually consume in one day, one or two quarts. Pour enough smoothie into a glass for your morning enjoyment and keep the rest in the refrigerator or another cold place, but not the freezer.

Sip your green smoothie slowly, mixing it with saliva for better absorption. Sometimes I put my smoothie in a coffee mug and carry it with me to the car or office. That way I minimize the chance of spilling it, and others don't notice the green contents of my cup.

Don't add anything to your smoothie except greens, fruit, and water. I don't recommend adding nuts, seeds, oils, supplements, or other ingredients to your green smoothie because most of these items slow down the assimilation of smoothies in your digestive tract and may cause irritation and gas. Even though I provide some recipes with these ingredients for special occasions in the book, I encourage you to stick to the basic green smoothie recipe (fruit and greens) in your daily routine.

Drink your smoothie by itself, and not as a part of a meal. To get the most nutritional benefits out of your green smoothie, don't consume anything, even as little as a cracker, with it. You can eat anything you want approximately forty minutes before or after your smoothie.

Do not add starchy vegetables such as carrots, beets, broccoli stems, zucchini, cauliflower, cabbage, Brussels sprouts, eggplant, pumpkin, squash, okra, peas, corn, and green beans to your green smoothies. Starchy vegetables combine poorly with fruit and may produce what my children call "gas-4-less."

Don't add too many ingredients to one smoothie, such as four different fruits and six different greens. To keep things easy on your digestive system, try to keep most of your recipes simple to maximize nutritional benefits.

Learn to prepare a really delicious green smoothie so that you are always looking forward to the next one. If your drink is not tasty, you will eventually give up on it. Keep your taste buds happy.

You should always rotate the green leaves that you add to your smoothies. Almost all greens in the world contain minute amounts of alkaloids. Tiny quantities of alkaloids cannot hurt you, and even strengthen the immune system. However, if you keep consuming kale, or spinach, or any other single green for many weeks without rotation, eventually the same type of alkaloids can accumulate in your body and cause unwanted symptoms of poisoning. (I discuss more of the significance of rotation of greens in Chapter 4.) Please note that you don't have to rotate the fruit in your green smoothies. Most commonly used fruits contain very few or no alkaloids and cannot cause the same toxic reactions as greens. However, rotating fruits will enhance the variety of flavor and nutrition in your smoothies.

Choose organic produce whenever possible. The absence of pesticides and other toxic chemicals is only one of the many benefits of organic food. The most important reason to consume organic food is the superior nutrition of organic fruits and vegetables in comparison to conventionally grown produce. Above, I discussed how nutritionally deficient most people are. The best way to nourish your body is to consume organic produce and, whenever possible, locally grown produce as well. I consider it very important to eat fruit that was allowed to fully ripen on the vine because it is several times more nutritious than unripe fruit. You derive those benefits most completely when you consume fruit shortly after it has been picked. Produce that is shipped from great distances may have a cheaper price tag, but it's harder on the environment and on our health.

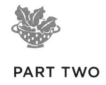

PART TWO

GREEN SMOOTHIE RECIPES

VALUABLE TIPS AND TRICKS FOR SMOOTHIE PREPARATION

YOU CAN USE ANY BLENDER TO MAKE SMOOTHIES, HOWEVER I recommend using the most powerful blender you can find, 1,000 watts or more. If you don't have a powerful blender, you can still make green smoothies and benefit from them, but you will have to chop your ingredients into smaller pieces, blend for longer periods of time, and put up with some chunks in your smoothie. A smoothie prepared in a high-speed blender is smooth in consistency and will be assimilated better by the body. For those who live in the United States, I recommend any model of the Vita-Mix blender. To purchase one free of shipping costs, visit my Web site at www.rawfamily.com. If you live outside of the United States, I recommend another high-speed blender, Blendtec, which is priced reasonably for international sales. To purchase this blender, visit www.thehealthylivingshow.com.

Blending time will depend on the ingredients you are using. I usually blend my smoothies for thirty seconds or less; however, when I blend hardy ingredients such as pomegranate seeds, celery, or slices of organic mango with peel, I might blend them for up to a minute. With tougher ingredients, I start at a low speed for approximately thirty seconds, then increase the speed and blend the smoothie until it is creamy, approximately another thirty seconds.

If you have a high-speed blender, we recommend not peeling organic fruit such as mangoes, apples, kiwis, and pears. You can also blend apples and pears with their seeds. If you have a regular blender that runs at slower speeds, peels and seeds will not blend completely and might destroy your blender. If you have a high-speed blender you can blend a pineapple's core but not the peel. We always peel fruit that is not organically grown.

Fruits that are rich in soluble fiber and pectin will make your smoothie creamy and will prevent the separation of liquid and fiber in the smoothie. My favorite fruits for smoothies are mangoes, bananas, pears, peaches, strawberries, and blueberries. The most likely cause of froth are apples, especially if they are not thoroughly blended. If you don't like the frothy appearance of your smoothie, here are some tips: Avocado pits have a high content of soluble fiber, so adding half of an avocado pit (seed) per 32 ounces of smoothie will reduce frothiness. However, only a high-speed blender can blend an avocado pit. For safety, cut the avocado pit while it is still inside of the avocado by slicing the entire fruit in half all the way through the middle. I usually add the avocado pit to my smoothie while its already blending to avoid wrecking the blender. You don't have to peel the avocado pit. Adding a whole avocado pit can result in a bitter-tasting smoothie. Another way of reducing froth is adding a cube or two of ice. Frothiness in your smoothie does not reduce its nutritional value, so you can simply shake it or stir it before drinking to reduce bubbles and separation.

You can blend greens whole, however I usually remove the stalks from kale, collards, and chard as they add a peppery taste that I don't like. I always leave the stalks on finer plants such as spinach, dandelions, parsley, and cilantro.

Several recipes call for coconut meat and water, so for those of you who are unfamiliar with coconut preparation, I include the following instructions below, excerpted with kind permission of Sergei and Valya Boutenko from their wonderful book *Fresh:*

> Young coconuts, which contain about 750 ml of water, are healthiest to eat. As the coconut matures, the soft jelly inside hardens into flesh and loses some nutritional qualities. To choose a good coconut, pick one up and give it a shake. If it's a good one, it will be heavy and completely filled with liquid. Because it has no air bubbles, you won't be able to hear the water splash around inside. Of the many ways to open a coconut, we believe it's best to begin by setting the coconut on its side. The

point (the top) should be pointing away from you. Take a large serrated knife and begin to shave the husk off of the point of the coconut so that the shell is revealed.

Rotate the coconut as needed and continue cutting off the husk all the way around the point. You will notice that under the white husk is a light brown shell. The coconuts usually seen in stores have their husk already removed. Make sure you have shaved off the husk in a complete circle so that it will be easier to open the coconut.

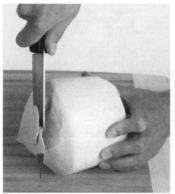
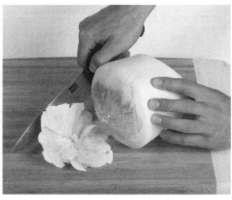

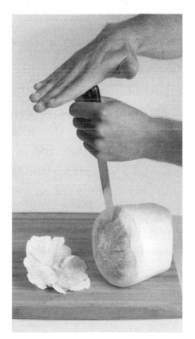

Place your knife just inside the circle you have shaved. Stab the knife into the shell. Coconut shells have a circular grain. When you force the knife through any part of the shell, a spherical crack will form. Cut about 1 inch into the shell of the coconut and slice down through the shell about 2 more inches.

Put the coconut pointed side up again so that the coconut water does not run out. Twist the knife slightly and a round opening will easily form at the top of the coconut. When the coconut top is half way separated from the rest of the shell, you can use your hands to help lift the top off completely.

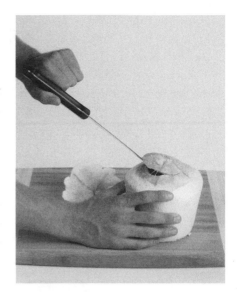

If you drink the water but don't want to eat the coconut meat right away, you may put the pointy shell top back on the coconut like a lid and store the coconut in the refrigerator for three or four days. To remove the coconut meat, use a spoon to scoop it out of the shell. The younger a coconut is, the thinner and softer the white meat will be. When the meat of a coconut is slightly pink, it means it is starting to ferment. In most cases, the coconut is still okay to eat, but both the meat and the water will taste different. If you have doubts, discard the coconut.

I anticipate that this book will be read by thousands of people in many different countries, where people use various measurements for fresh greens. To better explain the amounts of greens in the following smoothie recipes, I sometimes use cups and other times bunches as the unit of measurement. Do not be concerned about the varying sizes of bunches, as these recipes have plenty of room for error.

We have been collecting these recipes for four years from smoothie drinkers worldwide. We tried them all and selected only the best ones for your enjoyment.

GREEN SMOOTHIES FOR BEGINNERS

BASIC BALANCE
Victoria Boutenko

Yields 1 quart

     1 mango
     1 cup kale
     1 cup water

MORNING ZING SMOOTHIE
Victoria Boutenko

Yields 2 quarts

     ½ bunch dandelion greens
     2 stalks celery
     ½ inch fresh gingerroot
     2 peaches
     ½ pineapple

CANTALOUPE PARSLEY SMOOTHIE
Igor Boutenko

Yields 1 quart

     3 cups cantaloupe, cubed
     1 bunch fresh parsley

PARSLEY PASSION SMOOTHIE　　　Yields 2 quarts

Sergei Boutenko

>1 bunch fresh parsley
>1 cucumber, peeled
>1 Fuji apple
>1 ripe banana
>1–2 cups water

DANCING DANDELION SMOOTHIE

Igor Boutenko　　　Yields 2 quarts

>3 cups freshly picked dandelion greens
>2 cups apple juice
>1 cup water
>1 fresh mango
>1 ripe peach

DENT DE LION

Valya Boutenko　　　Yields 2 quarts

>1 bunch dandelion greens
>2 mangoes
>2 cups apple juice
>2 pears
>1 cup water

PERFECTLY PEACHY

Victoria Boutenko   **Yields 2 quarts**

3 peaches
1 head butter lettuce
½ pint raspberries
2 cups water

WICKED WATERMELON SMOOTHIE

Sergei Boutenko   **Yields 2 quarts**

4 cups fresh watermelon chunks,
    rind removed
1 banana
5 leaves romaine lettuce
Juice of ½ lemon

P-P-PAPAYA SMOOTHIE

Valya Boutenko   **Yields 1 quart**

2 cups spinach
1 fresh papaya, seeds removed
1 banana
1 cup water

MEDALLION MELON SMOOTHIE

Valya Boutenko   **Yields 1 quart**

3 cups cantaloupe, cubed
9 leaves romaine lettuce

EUROPEAN BLACK CURRANT SMOOTHIE

Yields 2 quarts

Victoria Boutenko

1 pint black currants
1 ripe mango
1 head butter lettuce
2 cups orange juice

THUNDERSTORM SMOOTHIE

Sergei Boutenko

Yields 2 quarts

1 cup pineapple chunks
1 cup star fruit chunks
1 cup pineapple guava chunks
1 banana
½ bunch chard
2 cups water

ROCKET FUEL SMOOTHIE

Victoria Boutenko

Yields 2 quarts

2 cups green or red seedless grapes
3 golden kiwis
1 ripe orange, peeled and seeded
1 small thumb-sized piece of aloe vera,
  with skin
5 leaves red leaf lettuce
2 cups water

MEMORY BOOSTER BRAIN SMOOTHIE

Valya Boutenko   **Yields 2 quarts**

> 2 cups freshly picked purslane
> 1 organic cucumber with peel
> 1 lime, ced
> 2 ripe pears
> ½ apple
> 2 cups water

ORIGINAL RAW FAMILY
SMOOTHIE IMPROVED

Victoria Boutenko   **Yields 2 quarts**

> 1 pint strawberries (fresh or frozen)
> 2 ripe bananas
> ½ avocado
> 2 cups water
> 4–6 leaves dinosaur kale

PINK AND GREEN

Bethany Einschlag   **Yields 2 quarts**

> 1 Pink Lady apple
> 1 large d'Anjou pear
> 5 ounces frozen strawberries
> 3 cups red kale

GOOSEBERRY CRUSH

Valya Boutenko   **Yields 2 quarts**

1 pint gooseberries
3 cups green oak leaf lettuce
2 cups apple juice

LOVELY GREEN GOODNESS

Tom Morrison   **Yields 2 quarts**

2 bananas
1 Royal Gala apple
1 Bosc pear
1 cup kale
¼ cup water

SWEET PARSLEY SMOOTHIE

Mieke Hays   **Yields 2 quarts**

2 cups fresh parsley
1 Fuji apple
1 banana
2 Medjool dates, pitted
2 ounces fresh lemon juice

GREENA COLADA

Kathy Stoner **Yields 2 quarts**

1 cup spinach
2 bananas
⅓ pineapple
½ cup coconut meat
1 cup coconut water

WINTER GREEN SMOOTHIE

Victoria Boutenko **Yields 2 quarts**

1 cup organic frozen berries (any kind)
2 cups fresh spinach
2 cups water
¼ inch fresh gingerroot, or to taste

Decorate with a slice of fruit.

GOJI BERRY ENCHANTMENT

Sergei Boutenko **Yields 2 quarts**

1 cup goji berries, soaked for 20 minutes
1 mango
3 tangerines, peeled and seeded
2 stalks celery
1 head butter lettuce
1 cup water

IMPEACHMINT!

Reni Atanassov   **Yields 1 quart**

> 1 ripe peach or ½ cup frozen peaches
> 1 sprig mint, or 5–7 mint leaves
> 1 cup spinach
> 1 cup water

ROMINTIC MANGO

Reni Atanassov   **Yields 1 quart**

> 1 ripe mango
> 1 cup romaine lettuce
> 1 sprig mint, or 5–7 mint leaves

APPLE GREEN SMOOTHIE

Anne Lebe   **Yields 2 quarts** r

> 4 cups romaine lettuce
> 4 Fuji apples
> ½ cup dates, pitted
> ¼ teaspoon cinnamon
> 3 cups water

SASKATOON SUNRISE

Theadora Leigh McBride   **Yields 2 quarts**

1 cup dandelion greens
1 cup fresh Italian parsley
2 bananas
2 cups Saskatoon berries (or blueberries)
2 cups water

LOVE POTION

Valya Boutenko   **Yields 2 quarts**

4 cups wild sorrel
4 cups fresh watermelon chunks, rind
  removed
4 ripe white nectarines
10 organically grown red rose petals
1 organically grown four-leaf clover
  (or 4 three-leaf clovers)

TROPICAL GREEN SMOOTHIE

Janice Snow   **Yields 2 quarts**

2 cups spinach
1 mango
1 banana
1 cup pineapple chunks
1 cup water

FAVORITE GREEN SMOOTHIE

Vanessa Nowitzky   **Yields 1 quart**

> 3–6 leaves any kind of kale, depending
> on how large the leaves are (keep the
> stems except for the hardest inch at
> the bottom)
> 1 banana
> 1 apple
> ½ inch fresh gingerroot
> 2 cups water

YUMMERIFIC!

Derrin and Helen Dallman and kids   **Yields 2 quarts**

> 2 cups dandelion greens
> 1–2 cups blackberries
> 2 cups tangelo juice
> 1 tablespoon honey (optional)

REVOLUTION-EVOLUTION

Babsi Clark   **Yields 2 quarts**

> 2 cups dinosaur kale
> 2–3 apples
> 1 Meyer lemon, peeled, seeds removed
> ½ inch fresh gingerroot
> 4 cups water
> ½ cup raisins (optional)

EVERY MORNING

Naomi Lorenzini   **Yields 2 quarts**

2 cups spinach
1 banana
2 cups orange juice
1 cup frozen blueberries
1 cup strawberries (optional)

BLUE SKIES GREEN SMOOTHIE

Pamela Nesbit   **Yields 2 quarts**

1 cup dandelion greens
1 cup fresh parsley
3 apples
1 cup blueberries
1 cup cranberries
2 cups water

I CAN'T BELIEVE IT'S GREEN SMOOTHIE

Esse Hopper   **Yields 2 quarts**

2 cups green chard
1–2 stalks celery
2 cups cherry tomatoes
1 ripe pear
1 Pink Lady apple
1 cup water

ANDREA'S GREEN DELIGHT

Samantha Johnson   **Yields 2 quarts**

2 cups spinach
1 green apple
1 yellow apple
2 bananas
3 cups water

GOOD STUFF

Margaret Miller   **Yields 2 quarts**

2 cups romaine lettuce
2 apples, peeled
2 pears
1 banana
Juice of ½ lemon
2 cups water

BLACK SHEEP

Eileen Young   **Yields 1 quart**

2 cups lambsquarters
4 figs
½ cup blueberries
2 cups water

CHRISTMAS IN JUNE

Chris Sabatini   **Yields 2 quarts**

> 2 cups spinach, packed
> 1 mango
> 2 oranges, peeled and seeded
> 2 sprigs fresh rosemary, leaves only

GREEN JULIUS

Charlene McClellan   **Yields 2 quarts**

> 1 ½ cups orange juice, freshly squeezed
> 2 cups ice
> 2 large mangoes
> 2 cups fresh parsley or spinach

TURKISH GROVE

Kristin Whitcoe   **Yields 2 quarts**

> 2 cups kale
> 1 d'Anjou pear
> 3 Turkish figs
> 2 cups water

CITRUS SUNLIGHT
Mary Ellis   **Yields 2 quarts**

1 apple
½ tangelo
½ nectarine
½ banana
1 teaspoon lemon juice
1 cup fresh parsley
1 cup water

FIG FANTASY
Reni Atanassov   **Yields 2 quarts**

6 figs
2 cups spinach, packed
1 sprig mint, or 4–6 leaves mint
1 cup water

PINEAPPLE SPICE CAKE
Marie-Noëlle Maltais   **Yields 2 quarts**

½ pineapple
1 mango
2 bananas
1 small piece fresh gingerroot
¼ teaspoon cinammon
¼ teaspoon nutmeg
1 cup chard, packed
1 cup water

RED GREEN SMOOTHIE

Saint Algie   **Yields 2 quarts**

> 2 cups red leaf lettuce, packed
> 2 nectarines
> 8 strawberries
> 1 cup water

RED SMOOTHIE

Jan Ektarian   **Yields 2 quarts**

> 1 apple
> ½ cup fresh parsley
> ½ cup cilantro
> 5 beet leaves, with stems
> 1 cup water

SUMMERTIME SMOOTHIE

Kathy Ramsey   **Yields 2 quarts**

> 1 cup beet greens
> 1 Fuji apple
> ½ banana
> ½ cup water

WINTER GREEN SMOOTHIE

Victoria Boutenko   **Yields 1 quart**

> 1 cup organic frozen berries (any kind)
> 2 cups fresh spinach greens
> 2 cups water
> ¼ inch fresh gingerroot, or to taste

Decorate with a slice of fruit.

SERGEI'S PARTY IN YOUR MOUTH GREEN SMOOTHIE

Sergei Boutenko   **Yields 2 quarts**

> 1 small pineapple
> 1 large mango, peeled
> ½ head romaine lettuce
> 1 sliver of fresh gingerroot, about the size
>   of half a pinky finger

WHEAT GRASS-HOPPER

Valya Boutenko   **Yields 1.5 quarts**

> 2 cups fresh-cut wheatgrass
> 1 mango
> 2 bananas
> 2 cups water

SUPERGREEN SMOOTHIES

VICTORIA'S FAVORITE DARK GREEN

Victoria Boutenko   **Yields 2 quarts**

> 1 bunch dandelion greens
> 4 Roma tomatoes
> 3 cups water

GREEN SMOOTHIE MONSTER

Victoria Boutenko   **Yields 2 quarts**

> 4 leaves kale
> 4 leaves chard
> ½ bunch fresh parsley
> 1 leaf aloe vera
> ½ bunch dandelion greens
> 3 pears
> 1 banana
> 3 cups water

DARK GREEN LOVE

Victoria Boutenko   **Yields 2 quarts**

1 bunch dandelion greens
1 medium cucumber
3 cups water

DOUBLE GREEN SMOOTHIE

Victoria Boutenko   **Yields 2 quarts**

1 bunch dandelion greens
1 bunch fresh parsley
1 cup fresh blueberries
1 pear
3 cups water

DANDY LIONS

Valya Boutenko   **Yields 1 quart**

1 bunch dandelion greens
3 cups apple juice
1 ripe mango

MIDSUMMER

Chris Sabatini   **Yields 2 quarts**

1 cup purslane, packed
1 cup fresh parsley, packed
2 oranges, peeled and seeded
1 grapefruit, peeled and seeded
1 mango
1 cup water

ANTICANCER SMOOTHIE

Victoria Boutenko   **Yields 1 quart**

1 pint broccoli sprouts
1 pint ripe organic blackberries
1 cup water

PRICKLY ANTICANCER RECIPE

Victoria Boutenko   **Yields 2 quarts**

3 cups milk thistle
1 apple
1 pint strawberries
2 cups black seedless grapes
2 cups knotweed
2 cups water

GREEN JUNGLE JAMBOREE

Valya Boutenko   **Yields 2 quarts**

4 cups mallow (also known as *Malva*)
4 cups miner's lettuce
2 cups chickweed
1 banana
5 golden kiwis
1 papaya
2 cups water

FOR THE BRAVE

Igor Boutenko   **Yields 2 quarts**

1 cup carrot tops
1 cup beet greens
1 cup bok choy
½ cup horsetail
1 cup plums
1 banana
4 kiwis
2 cups water

RESVERATROL ELIXIR OF LIFE

Victoria Boutenko   **Yields 1 quart**

4 cups knotweed
5 young grape leaves (they contain resveratrol, which triggers longevity genes)
2 mangoes
2 cups water

VITAMIN C MASTER COMBO

Victoria Boutenko   **Yields 1 quart**

> 4 cups miner's lettuce
> 2 cups sorrel
> Juice of ½ lemon
> 2 pears
> 2 cups water

SPICY SINUS CLEANSER

Igor Boutenko   **Yields 2 quarts**

> 1 cup fresh watercress
> 1 small leaf horseradish
> 1 cucumber
> ¼-inch slice chili pepper
> 1 large tomato
> 2 stalks celery
> Juice of 1 lemon
> 1 cup water

HEAVY METALS BE GONE

Valya Boutenko   **Yields 2 quarts**

> 1 bunch cilantro
> 2 cups stinging nettles
> 1 bunch fresh parsley
> 3 stalks celery
> Juice of 1 lemon
> 2 mangoes
> 2 cups apple juice

WORLD'S SAFEST LIVER CLEANSER

Victoria Boutenko   **Yields 2 quarts**

4 cups fresh dandelion greens and blossoms
½ head endive
2 cups milk thistle
2 cups apple juice
1 banana
2 pears
1 inch fresh gingerroot
1 cup cranberries

CHICKEN SCRATCH

Gabrielle Chavez   **Yields 1 quart**

2 cups chickweed
2 cups mâche
4 pears
2 cups water

GREEN STINGER

Gabrielle Chavez   **Yields 2 quarts**

4 cups grapes
2 slices lemon, with peel, seeds removed
4 cups stinging nettle tops
2-inch piece aloe vera
1–2 cups water

DAILY MEAL

Irene   **Yields 2 quarts**

4 cups spinach
1 banana
3 medium tomatoes
3 cups water

SATISFYING SMOOTHIE

Victoria Boutenko   **Yields 2 quarts**

1 bunch kale
1 bunch chard
3 red bell peppers, with seeds, stems
  removed
3 cups water

PURSLANE GREEN SMOOTHIE

Victoria Boutenko   **Yields 1 quart**

4 cups purslane
4 ripe peaches
2 cups water
1 cup ice

CACTUS GREEN SMOOTHIE

Ed   **Yields 1 quart**

> 2 large nopal cactus paddles, with thorns
> 1 cup green grapes

STINGING NETTLE GREEN SMOOTHIE

Victoria Boutenko   **Yields 1 quart**

> ½ cup stinging nettle leaves
> 1 mango
> 1 tablespoon lemon juice
> 2 cups water

SIMPLY DELICIOUS
DOUBLE-GREEN PUDDING

Victoria Boutenko   **Yields 2 quarts**

> 1 bunch dandelion greens
> 1 pint blueberries
> 1 cup water

VELVET GREEN SMOOTHIE

Victoria Boutenko   **Yields 2 quarts**

> 1 bunch dandelion greens
> 1 bunch parsley
> 3 mangoes
> 3 cups water

SAVORY GREEN SMOOTHIES AND SOUPS

MEDITERRANEAN SOUP

Victoria Boutenko   **Yields 3 quarts**

3 cups spinach
3 stalks celery
1 sprig oregano
1 sprig thyme
1 red bell pepper
1 large avocado
1 cucumber
1 jalapeño pepper
1 lime, juiced
2 cups water

Enjoy with dulse leaves or flakes.

CUCUMBER DILL-ICIOUS SOUP

Valya Boutenko   **Yields 2 quarts**

2 cucumbers
½ bunch dill
1 large avocado
5 leaves dinosaur kale
2 stalks celery
1 lime, juiced
3 cloves garlic

OREGANO TUMMY SOOTHER

Igor Boutenko   **Yields 3 cups**

1 sprig oregano
1 sprig rosemary
½ avocado
1 cucumber
2 cups mallow (also known as *Malva*)

SOUP GAZPACHO

Victoria Boutenko   **Yields 2 quarts**

3 leaves kale
1 bunch basil
3 large tomatoes
2 stalks celery
1 red bell pepper
1 large avocado
1 lime, juiced
1 cup water
2 cups love

THAI SOUP

Sergei Boutenko   **Yields 2 quarts**

2 cucumbers

1 large avocado

Juice of 1 lime

3 cloves garlic

6 leaves curly kale

½ inch fresh turmeric root (or ½ teaspoon
    dried turmeric powder)

½ inch fresh gingerroot (or ¼ teaspoon
    dried ginger powder)

2 cups water

NEIGHBOR'S GARDEN

Sergei Boutenko   **Yields 1 quart**

2 cups pumpkin or squash leaves

1 small zucchini

6 cherry tomatoes

8 snap peas

½ bunch fresh dill (or any other herb you
    can find)

1 cup turnip greens

½ cup carrot tops

Juice of 1 lime

1 avocado

2 cups water

MUSTARD MUSKETEER

Valya Boutenko   **Yields 1 quart**

> 1 cup fresh mustard leaves and blossoms
> 1 large avocado
> 3 pickling cucumbers
> 1 bunch baby bok choy
> Juice of 1 lemon
> 2 cups water

Blend and pour into a large bowl. Stir in remaining ingredients:

> 1 carrot, grated
> 1 cup bok choy, chopped
> 3 calendula flowers
> ½ avocado, cubed
> 2 pickling cucumbers, sliced
> ¼ cup dulse leaves

ALL KINDS OF PEPPERS AND TOMATOES

Victoria Boutenko   **Yields 2 quarts**

> 1 large avocado
> 1 yellow bell pepper
> 1 red bell pepper
> 1 medium tomato
> 3 cups baby greens (no arugula)
> 1 bunch cilantro
> Juice of 1 lime
> 2 cups water

SAVORY BASIL SOUP

Valya Boutenko   **Yields 1 quart**

1 bunch fresh basil
2 large ripe tomatoes
1 bell pepper, seeds and stem removed
2 cloves garlic
1 cup water

Blend and pour into a large bowl. Stir in remaining ingredients:

3 cups Savoy cabbage, chopped
3 green onions, sliced
½ cup dulse
½ avocado, cubed

GARDEN WALK

Fiona Blasius   **Yields 1 quart**

1 cup baby spinach, packed
1 cup fresh parsley, packed
2 medium tomatoes
2 tablespoons lemon juice
¼ jalapeño pepper, or to taste
½ avocado

SPICY GREEN SOUP

Victoria Boutenko **Yields 1 quart**

2 cups spinach
1 cup radish tops (or mustard greens,
    horseradish greens, watercress,
    or other spicy greens)
½ cup fresh basil
1 red bell pepper
2 limes, peeled
2 medium-size ripe tomatoes
½ avocado
2 cups water

Serve as soup with dulse or any other seaweed.

COOL SUMMER SMOOTHIE

Leslie DeLorean **Yields 2 quarts**

½ bunch fresh parsley
1 cucumber
½ bunch dill
½ avocado
½ lemon, peeled, seeds removed
2 cups water

JIM'S BASIC BASIL

Jim Tibbetts **Yields 1 quart**

2 tomatoes
2 stalks celery
1 cup spinach, packed
½ cup fresh basil

SAVORY CUCUMBER LASSI

Renate and Steve Behrens **Yields 1 quart**

2 cucumbers
1 lemon, peeled
2 celery stalks
1 avocado
1 mango

FENNEL SOUP

Niz Marar **Yields 2 quarts**

2 cups kale
2 stalks celery
1 stalk fennel
½ avocado
½ lemon
2 cups water
¼ inch turmeric root (optional)

LIVER LOVER

Mindy Goldis   **Yields 2 quarts**

2 cups dandelion greens
2 stalks celery
1 cup fresh parsley
1 green zucchini
1 ½ d'Anjou pears
½ teaspoon fresh gingerroot
½ teaspoon turmeric
1 dash cayenne pepper
1 teaspoon lemon juice

BOK CHOY JOY

Mindy Goldis   **Yields 2 quarts**

2 cups bok choy
½ cup fresh cilantro
½ zucchini squash
1 stalk celery
1 apple
¼ teaspoon fresh gingerroot
¼ teaspoon fresh turmeric
1 dash lemon juice
1 pinch cayenne pepper

MORNING GLORY

Julie Roberts   **Yields 2 quarts**

¼ jalapeño pepper
1 ½ cups kale
2 medium oranges, peeled and seeded
1 clove garlic
½ teaspoon fresh gingerroot
½ cup cilantro

ONE TOUGH BANANA

Jo Ridgway   **Yields 1 quart**

1 banana
½ cup kale
1 small clove garlic
½ cup water

WHAT A PAIR!

Dianne Marshall   **Yields 3 cups**

2 medium Bartlett pears, peeled, stems
    removed
½ cup fennel fronds
½ cup water

HERB GARDEN

Mindy Goldis   **Yields 2 quarts**

½ cup kale
1 cucumber
1 tomato
1 avocado
2 stalks fennel
¼ cup basil
¼ cup oregano
½ cup water
2 tablespoons lemon juice

RADICAL RADISH

Mindy Goldis   **Yields 2 quarts**

1 cup radish greens
1 stalk celery
½ stalk fennel
1 pear
1 thin slice fresh gingerroot
1 thin slice turmeric
1 pinch cayenne pepper
1 tablespoon lemon juice
½ tablespoon flaxseeds

DILLY CRAZY BABY BOK CHOY

Marie-Noëlle Maltais **Yields 1 quart**

1 bunch baby bok choy
¼ cup fresh dill
2 tablespoons lemon juice
½ teaspoon stevia
½ cup water

REFRESHING CUCUMBER SPINACH

Cheryl Leghorn **Yields 1 quart**

1 cucumber
1 cup spinach, packed
2 tablespoons lime juice
1 teaspoon honey
1 sprig spearmint, or 5–7 spearmint leaves
½ cup water

IMMUNE BOOSTER

Kathy Ramsey **Yields 1 quart**

½ cucumber
¼ leek
½ cup radish sprouts
1 clove garlic
4 tablespoons lemon juice
1 cup water
1 avocado

MANGO TARRAGON

Marie-Noëlle Maltais   **Yields 1 quart**

> 2 mangoes
> 3–4 leaves tarragon
> 4 tablespoons lemon juice
> 2 cups chard
> 1 cup water

RABBIT PATCH

Chris Sabatini   **Yields 1 quart**

> 2 medium tomatoes
> 1 cucumber
> ½ cup carrot tops
> ½ sugar baby watermelon, or two cups
>   chopped
> 1 cup kale

SPINACH COLD BUSTER

Vanessa Nowitzky   **Yields 2 quarts**

> 2 cups spinach
> 12 cloves garlic
> Juice of 1 lemon
> ½ cucumber (add more if it's too hot)
> ¼ teaspoon cayenne pepper
> ½ teaspoon minced jalapeño pepper
> 1 cup water

ORANGE AID

Vanessa Nowitzky   **Yields 2 quarts**

2 cups arugula
½ orange bell pepper
2 oranges, peeled and seeded
1 clove garlic
1 jalapeño pepper
1 dash cayenne pepper, or to taste

Blend and pour into a bowl. Add ½ avocado in chunks.

PROBIOTIC GUACAMOLE SPREAD

Igor Boutenko   **Yields 3 cups**

1 cup sauerkraut
2 large avocados
3 tablespoons lemon juice
1 cup spinach
1 cup fresh dill

SCARLET HONEY MUSTARD SPREAD

Valya Boutenko   **Yields 2 cups**

1 cup fresh mustard greens
1 cup beet greens
1 avocado
½ beet
Juice of ½ lime

CELERY SOUP

Dena Garrison   **Yields 2 quarts**

1 cup fresh parsley
4 stalks celery
1 avocado
½ cup olive oil
Juice of 1 lemon
1 tomato
1 tablespoon honey
¼ teaspoon sea salt
3 cups water

CELERY ZING SOUP

Chris Sabatini   **Yields 1 quart**

2 yellow bell peppers
1 lemon
½ cup basil leaves
1 cup celery, tops and greens
1 cup dinosaur kale
1 cup water

ORANGE ZEST

Vanessa Nowitzky   **Yields 1 quart**

2 cups arugula
½ orange bell pepper
2 oranges, peeled and seeded
1 banana (optional to make it sweeter,
    but it's already pretty sweet!)

PURPLE GREEN SMOOTHIE

Michèle Moisan   **Yields 1 quart**

> 2 cups fresh Italian parsley
> 1 cup blueberries
> 1 cup red grapes
> 1 cucumber

RAW FAMILY GREEN SOUP

Victoria Boutenko   **Yields 1 quart**

> 3 leaves chard
> 1 stalk celery
> ½ bunch fresh parsley
> Juice of 1 lemon
> 1 large avocado
> 2 cups water

Add water as needed and blend to a desired consistency. We like to add dulse leaves, grated carrots, grated cauliflower, and sprouts to our bowl of soup.

SWEET SOUP

Valya Boutenko   **Yields 2 quarts**

> 1 bunch dill
> 4 stalks celery
> 2 apples
> 1 lemon, peeled
> 1 avocado, peeled and seeded
> 2 cups water

GREEN SMOOTHIES
FOR ADVENTUROUS SOULS

SUMMER SPLENDOR SMOOTHIE

Sergei Boutenko **Yields 2 quarts**

4 leaves chard
3 stalks celery
1 bunch fresh parsley
6 apricots
3 peaches
½ vanilla bean

O-MEGA APHRODISIAC

Victoria Boutenko **Yields 2 quarts**

3 cups wild purslane
1 small watermelon, with rind
Juice of 3 limes

REVITALIZING ENERGIZER SMOOTHIE

Victoria Boutenko   **Yields 1 quart**

6 young grape leaves (they contain resveratrol, which triggers longevity genes)

3 leaves dinosaur kale

2 mangoes

1 pint strawberries

2 cups orange juice

FOREST FULL OF TREES

Chris Sabatini   **Yields 2 quarts**

1 cup dandelion greens, packed

1 cup spinach, packed

2 cups strawberries

3 mangoes

¼ cup pine needles

2 cups water

"BITTER DELIGHT" COCKTAIL

Victoria Boutenko   **Yields 1 quart**

1 large leaf aloe vera, with skin

4 leaves chard

3 cups chickweed

1 banana

1 peach

1 pear

BLEH! "SO BLAND, WHY DID I TRY THIS, BUT IT'S GROWING ON ME" SMOOTHIE

Valya Boutenko   **Yields 2 quarts**

3 cups buckwheat sprouts, hulls removed

1 cup frisée lettuce

1 cup green table grapes

1 banana

1 pear

1 avocado seed (a wonderful source of soluble fiber)

2 cups apple juice

SEA BUCKTHORN RUMBA

Victoria Boutenko   **Yields 1 quart**

½ cup sea buckthorn berries

1 cup goji leaves (we grow these from goji berries)

2 plums

1 apple

1 banana

1 cup water

1 stalk celery

HONEYDEW & DANDELION

Victoria Boutenko   **Yields 2 quarts**

1 honeydew melon, peeled, seeds removed

1 large bunch dandelion greens

TOOTY FRUITY

Valya Boutenko   **Yields 1 quart**

> 1 cup jackfruit
> 1 mango
> 2 cups baby bok choy
> 1 cup water

OH BAY-BEH BAY-BEH

Sergei Boutenko   **Yields 1 quart**

> 1 cup borage, leaves and flowers
> 4 kiwis
> 1 banana
> 1 cup water

WILD MELON SMOOTHIE

Victoria Boutenko   **Yields 2 quarts**

> 1 cantaloupe, peeled, seeds removed
> 5 cups lambsquarters

APHRODISIAC COCKTAIL

Victoria Boutenko   **Yields 2 quarts**

> 1 whole washed organic watermelon, with
> seeds and rind

PRICKLY PEAR GREEN-GO

Sergei Boutenko   **Yields 1 quart**

4 prickly pears, peeled
3 cups chard
1 banana
1 small apple
2 cups water

POMPOUS PERSIMMON COCKTAIL

Valya Boutenko   **Yields 1 quart**

2 ripe persimmons
1 large ripe pear
¼ bunch fresh mint
2 cups water

HAWAIIAN HIBISCUS

Sergei Boutenko   **Yields 3 cups**

1 cup hibiscus leaves
1 young coconut, meat and water
¼ pineapple

SILLY CILANTRO

Igor Boutenko   **Yields 1 quart**

1 bunch cilantro
3 pears
3 apricots
3 cups water

MORNING SPARK

Fiona Blasius   **Yields 1 quart**

1 cup arugula, packed
¼ pineapple
1 banana
¼ cup water

PEACHY KEEN GREEN

Carolyn Agee   **Yields 1 quart**

2 ripe organic peaches (or 10 ounces frozen
    peaches)
1 grapefruit, juiced
1 cup green kale
¾ cup water

WILD GREEN PEAR

Ryan and Crystal Fisk   **Yields 1 quart**

> 1 Bartlett pear
> 1 cup wild local greens
> 1 cup water

GREEN CAPRICE

Chris Sabatini   **Yields 1 quart**

> 1 mango
> 1 kiwi
> 1 cup collard greens, stems removed
> 2 strawberries
> 1 sprig basil
> 1 cup water

GREEN STAR

Aldo Aragao   **Yields 2 quarts**

> 1 pear
> ½ cup sunflower sprouts
> ½ cup chard
> ½ cup fresh parsley
> 3 tablespoons lime juice
> 1 leaf aloe vera, with skin
> ½ cup water
> 2 ice cubes

FRUITY WEEDS

Celeste Crimi   **Yields 2 quarts**

> 3 Valencia oranges, peeled and seeded
> ½ cup raspberries
> 1 cup lambsquarters
> ½ cup water
> ½ teaspoon stevia leaves
> 4 ice cubes

TODAY'S DISCOVERY

Janita Ielasi   **Yields 2 quarts**

> 4 bananas, peeled and frozen
> 3 small leaves aloe vera, with skin
> 2 cups celery tops
> ¼ cup chocolate mint leaves
> ½ cup water

SWEET TART SMOOTHIE

Mieke Hays   **Yields 2 quarts**

> 1 cup collard greens, stems removed
> ½ cup alfalfa sprouts
> ½ pineapple
> 1 banana
> 3 Medjool dates, pitted
> 3 tablespoons lemon juice
> 1 cup water

STEVEN'S TROPICAL WIGMORE-INSPIRED ENERGY SMOOTHIE

Steven Prussack   **Yields 2 quarts**

1 cup kale or chard
1 cup sunflower sprouts
¼ pineapple
1 mango
1 banana
1 cup water

ANTIOXIDANT LONGEVITY SMOOTHIE

Victoria Boutenko   **Yields 1 quart**

1 cup pomegranate seeds
1 cup spinach
1 cup water

SPRINGTIME DOUGLAS FIR SMOOTHIE

Victoria Boutenko   **Yields 1 quart**

10 new-growth, light-green tips of Douglas
    Fir needles
2 cups spinach
2 bananas
1 apple
2 cups water

BLOODY MARY

Leslie DeLorean   **Yields 1 quart**

½ bunch (or 1 cup) fresh parsley
3 stalks celery
3 Roma tomatoes
½ lemon, peeled, seeds removed
½ cup water
2 tablespoons dulse flakes

You can add a few shakes of cayenne pepper to add heat.

HOT STUFF

Leslie DeLorean   **Yields 1 quart**

1 bunch lambsquarters
2 red bell peppers, seeds removed
2 stalks celery
½ avocado
½ jalapeño pepper—if you can handle it
1 cup water

GREEN SMOOTHIE WITH MINER'S LETTUCE

Sergei Boutenko   **Yields 1 quart**

5 cups fresh miner's lettuce
1 ripe mango
1 apple
2 cups water

GREEN PUDDINGS

Puddings enrich the diversity of textures and flavors you can enjoy in green smoothies. Puddings are thicker smoothies that you can eat with a spoon. Green puddings generally don't contain any water and are often thickened with chia seeds, dates, coconut, mangoes, or blueberries. We recommend using a tamper, which often comes packaged with blenders, to help mix these thicker smoothies as you blend.

PERSIMMON PUDDING

Victoria Boutenko   **Yields 2 cups**

> 3 Furyu persimmons, peeled, seeds removed
> 3 cups baby spinach
> 1 ripe banana

THE PEAR-FECT SMOOTHIE

Katya Gladkikh   **Yields 2 cups**

> 2 d'Anjou pears
> 7 leaves purple kale
> 1 leaf aloe vera
> 1 banana

KENT MANGO BLISS

Victoria Boutenko   **Yields 3 cups**

>   2 Kent mangoes
>   1 bunch chard
>   1 pear
>   1 banana

Serve with kiwi.

GREEN PUDDING

Victoria Boutenko   **Yields 2 cups**

>   1 bunch fresh parsley
>   5 grape leaves
>   ½ pineapple
>   1 Abbot pear
>   1 orange, peeled and seeded
>   1 cup water

APPLESAUCE

Valya Boutenko   **Yields 3 cups**

>   4 apples
>   1 banana
>   1 head romaine lettuce
>   ½ teaspoon cinnamon
>   2 cups water

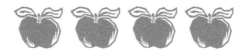

MANGO-LIME PUDDING

Sergei Boutenko   **Yields 2 cups**

2 ripe mangoes, peeled
2 cups chard
1 ripe banana
½ lime, with peel

BLUEBERRY ZING

Julie Rodwell   **Yields 2 cups**

1 cup fresh parsley, packed
1 small piece fresh gingerroot
1 orange, peeled and seeded
½ cup blueberries

SHELAH'S TANGY PUDDING

Shelah Segal   **Yields 2 cups**

½ pineapple
1 banana
2 kiwis
2 stalks celery
5 leaves dinosaur kale

PAPAYAVOCADO PUDDING

Mieke Hays   **Yields 2 cups**

1 papaya
1 small avocado
1 cup spinach

SPLENDID CALENDULA

Victoria Boutenko **Yields 2 cups**

½ cup fresh calendula greens
1 apple
2 peaches

MELLOW MALLOW

Sergei Boutenko **Yields 2 cups**

3 cups mallow (also known as *Malva*)
½ honeydew melon, peeled, seeds removed
1 mango

RED BANDIT

Valya Boutenko **Yields 2 cups**

1 cup beet greens
1 cup cranberries (fresh or frozen)
5 Medjool dates, pitted
1 banana
1 blood orange, peeled and seeded

LEMON PUDDING

Valya Boutenko   **Yields 2 cups**

> 1 banana
> 1 mango
> Juice of ½ lemon
> 1 sprig lemon balm
> 1 cup spinach
> 1 teaspoon lemon zest

AVO-COCO PUDDING

Marie-Noëlle Maltais   **Yields 3 cups**

> 1 young coconut, meat and water
> 3 tablespoons lime juice
> 2 bananas
> 1 avocado
> 1 cup cilantro, packed
> 1 stalk celery

DURIAN GREEN PUDDING

Victoria Boutenko   **Yields 3 cups**

> 3 pieces durian, seeds removed
> 2 cups spinach
> 1 banana

LAMBSQUARTERS OMEGA PUDDING

Victoria Boutenko · Yields 3 cups

1 young coconut, meat and water
1 pint blueberries
3 cups lambsquarters
1 cup purslane
2 pears

VALYA'S GREEN PUDDING

Valya Boutenko · Yields 3 cups

½ pineapple
1 apple
1 pear
3 cups chard
1 sprig lemon balm

STRAWBERRY CRÈME

Paula Gipson · Yields 3 cups

1 cup coconut milk
1 tablespoon honey
1 cup strawberries (frozen or fresh)
½ cup cashews
1 cup romaine lettuce, firmly packed
1 tablespoon flaxseeds

CILANTRO SPARKLE

Aletha Nowitzky   **Yields 2 cups**

> 1 bunch cilantro
> 1 mango
> 1 orange, peeled and seeded

COLON SURPRISE PUDDING

Victoria Boutenko   **Yields 3 cups**

> 1 cup soaked prunes
> 1 bunch fresh parsley
> 1 banana
> 1 orange, peeled and seeded
> 1 apple
> ¼ teaspoon pumpkin pie spice (nutmeg and cinnamon)
> 3 tablespoons psyllium husk

Add psyllium husk last, after the all other ingredients have been blended thoroughly. Add psyllium through the top of the lid while the blender is still running. Once the psyllium is added, the smoothie will thicken quickly, so have containers ready to empty the blender contents into.

SWEET AND SALTY STAR PUDDING

Victoria Boutenko   **Yields 2 cups**

> 2 star fruit
> 1 cup chard
> 2 finger bananas

SUN GREEN PUDDING

Chris Sabatini   **Yields 2 cups**

2 cups kale
½ cup raisins, soaked overnight
2 bananas
1 kiwi
1 Medjool date, pitted

SUNLIGHT ON SOIL

Chris Sabatini   **Yields 2 cups**

1 mango
1 leaf aloe vera, with skin
½ cup raisins, soaked overnight
1 sprig mint, or 5–7 mint leaves
¼ cup cilantro
2 cups spinach

BANACADO

Clare Sabatini   **Yields 2 cups**

3 bananas
1 avocado
1 cup kale
1 cup water (or less, as desired)
2–3 Medjool dates, pitted

COCONUT CHAMELEON

Melanie Ellingsen   **Yields 2 cups**

1 young coconut, water and meat
2 bananas
1 cup strawberries
2 cups greens (dandelion, arugula, or parsley recommended)

DREAMSICLE SMOOTHIE

Vanessa Nowitzky   **Yields 2 cups**

2 stalks celery
2 bananas, peeled and frozen
6 strawberries or ½ cup blueberries (frozen or fresh)
2 cups coconut water

THREE-COURSE MEAL

Marian Frank   **Yields 3 cups**

1 cup baby spinach
8 leaves romaine lettuce
2 dates, pitted
1 tablespoon sunflower seeds, soaked overnight
1 tablespoon sesame seeds, soaked overnight
1 banana
1 cup water
1–2 ounces lemon juice

RECETTE DES CHAMPS CONGELÉS

Madeleine Laurendeau   **Yields 2 cups**

2 cups red lettuce
6 apples
2 cups frozen berries (any kind)
2 cups water

PERSIMMON GREEN SMOOTHIE

Victoria Boutenko   **Yields 2 cups**

5 ripe persimmons
5 leaves romaine lettuce
2 cups water

COCONUT DREAM PUDDING

Valya Boutenko   **Yields 2 quarts**

1 bunch chard
1 young coconut, meat and water
5 Medjool dates, pitted
2 apples
1 banana

SPINACH PUDDING

Victoria Boutenko **Yields 2 quarts**

2 bunches spinach
2 bananas
1 apple
1 mango
½ lemon with peel
2 tablespoons chia seeds
1 cup water

PINEAPPLE PUDDING WALTZ

Valya Boutenko **Yields 2 quarts**

1 pound baby greens salad mix
2 apples
1 pineapple
2 pears

DOUBLE GREEN PUDDING

Victoria Boutenko **Yields 1.5 quarts**

1 bunch spinach
1 head romaine lettuce
1 pint strawberries

GREEN SMOOTHIES FOR CHILDREN

COCO-TANGO

Sergei Boutenko   **Yields 2 quarts**

> 1 Thai coconut, meat and water
> 5 leaves kale
> 2 nectarines
> 2 peaches
> 1 mango

THE LAUGHING GORILLA

Valya Boutenko   **Yields 2 quarts**

> ½ head romaine lettuce
> 2 ripe bananas, peeled and frozen
> 2 oranges, peeled and seeded
> 1 mango
> 2 cups water

*Warning: consumption of smoothie may result in spontane-
ously occurring, extremely contagious gorilla laughter.*

MINER'S LETTUCE SMOOTHIE

Sergei Boutenko   **Yields 2 quarts**

3 cups wild crafted miner's lettuce (wild
    edible)
2 ripe pears
½ pint blueberries
2 cups water

FROZEN MANGO MINT

Sergei Boutenko   **Yields 2 quarts**

1 cup frozen mango chunks
1 cup water
½ cup fresh or frozen strawberries
½ bunch fresh mint
½ cup apple juice

BERRY BLUE SMOOTHIE

Victoria Boutenko   **Yields 2 quarts**

2–3 cups water
1 cup fresh or frozen blueberries
1 cup fresh or frozen blackberries
1 ripe pear
½ bunch purple kale

EMERALD APPLESAUCE

Aletha Nowitzky   **Yields 3 cups**

5 apples
1 bunch fresh parsley
½ inch fresh gingerroot

GRANDIOSE GRAPE SMOOTHIE

Stephan Boutenko   **Yields 2 quarts**

3 cups green or red seedless grapes
2 pears
2 cups water
1 banana
5–7 leaves beet greens

SMOOTHIE OF SUCCESS

Igor Boutenko   **Yields 2 quarts**

7 strawberries
2 pears
4 pineapple guavas
3 cups spinach
3 cups water

PINEAPPLE SPIN

Jo Ridgway   **Yields 1 quart**

1 cup spinach
¼ pineapple

MELLOW CRICKET

Cricket Lott **Yields 1 quart**

2 cups sunflower sprouts
½ pineapple

MULBERRY MAGIC

Valya Boutenko **Yields 2 quarts**

1 pint mulberries
1 ripe peach
2 cups spinach
2 cups water

RASPBERRY GUAVA MINT SWIRL

Sergei Boutenko **Yields 2 quarts**

1 pint raspberries
4 pineapple guavas
¼ bunch mint
5 leaves romaine lettuce
2 cups water

APRICOT NECTAR

Stephan Boutenko **Yields 2 quarts**

5 apricots
1 banana
1 bunch fresh parsley
3 cups water

OH, MY, WHAT'D YA PUT IN HERE? I CAN'T BELIEVE THIS IS GOOD FOR ME! SMOOTHIE

Marina Gadkikh   **Yields 2 quarts**

2 ripe mangoes, peeled
1 ripe peach
8 leaves romaine lettuce
3 cups water

CLEMENTINE CITRUS CIRCUS

Valya Boutenko   **Yields 2 quarts**

6 clementines, peeled
2 ripe bananas, peeled and frozen
1 cup curly kale
1 cup spinach

PURPLE TEETH MASQUERADE
(ALSO KNOWN AS DENTIST'S NIGHTMARE SMOOTHIE)

Valya Boutenko   **Yields 2 quarts**

1 pint blackberries
1 ripe banana
1 mango
7 leaves dinosaur kale
2 cups water

SWEET AND SOUR

Marian Fanok **Yields 2 quarts**

1 banana
1 cup frozen raspberries
8 leaves romaine lettuce
½ cup baby spinach
2 Medjool dates, pitted
¾ cup water

SPINACH FRESHNESS

Stephen Frketic **Yields 2 quarts**

1 orange, peeled and seeded
1 banana
4 frozen strawberries
1 cup spinach, packed
¼ cup water

GREEN MONKEY FACE

Julia Holt **Yields 1 quart**

1 young coconut, meat and water
1 orange, peeled and seeded
2 cups baby spinach

GREEN SMOOTHIE POPSICLES!

Pattie Lacefield **Yields 2 quarts**

2 cups spinach
2 cups frozen berries (any kind)
2 bananas
1 cup water

Pour into popsicle holders and freeze.

COCO-NASH SMOOTHIE

Michèle Moisan **Yields 1 quart**

2 cups spinach
1 avocado
1 coconut, meat and water
½ teaspoon vanilla

GREEN STRAWBERRY DRINK

Mary Ellis **Yields 2 quarts**

3 stalks celery
2 bananas
2 cups frozen strawberries
1 pear
2 cups water

DELICIOUS SPRING GREEN SMOOTHIE

Igor Boutenko   **Yields 1 quart**

5 cups miner's lettuce
6 Medjool dates, pitted
2 cups water

GREEN SMOOTHIES FOR PETS

As discussed in "Green Smoothies for our Pets" (see pp. 41–44), your cats and dogs will love green smoothies. Some pets will take to smoothies right away, others after a gradual introduction. We serve our cat about 2–3 tablespoons twice a week. Servings for dogs will vary between 2 tablespoons and 1 cup two to three times a week, depending on the size of your dog. Any extra smoothie mixture you've made will keep in the refrigerator for up to three days.

POOCHIE'S GOURMET GREEN SMOOTHIE

Yields 1 doggy bowl (1 cup)

1 cup kale
1 banana
1 cup water
2 tablespoons olive oil
1 teaspoon kelp (granules or powder)

FIDO'S DREAM

Yields 1 doggy bowl (1 cup)

1 cup spinach

1 apple

1 cup water

2 tablespoons olive oil

2 capsules fish oil (pour on the smoothie, in the bowl)

Add some torn nori sheets; dogs love it!

FLUFFY'S DELIGHT

Yields approximately 10 servings

1 cup wheatgrass clippings (or any other grass, not sprayed)

1 cup water

2 tablespoons olive oil

2 capsules fish oil (pour on the smoothie, in the bowl)

Pinch of catnip (optional)

You can freeze it in an ice-cube tray and serve it by the cube.

GREEN SMOOTHIES FOR BODY CARE

ALOE FACIAL CLEANSER

Valya Boutenko

Yields 1 cup

½ cucumber
½ avocado
1 large leaf aloe vera, with skin

Apply on skin as a sunscreen, or after sunburn, or to improve overall skin health. Keep on skin 10–30 minutes, then rinse off.

PLANTAIN SKIN SMOOTHIE

Sergei Boutenko

Yields 2 cups

3–4 cups freshly picked plantain
(wild edible)
1 cup water

Apply on skin to alleviate pain from bug bites, plant stings, rashes, and to improve overall skin quality. Great for eczema and acne.

AFTERWORD
THE WORLDWIDE GREEN SMOOTHIE REVOLUTION

Every generation needs a new revolution. —THOMAS JEFFERSON

At times I feel as if I let some old, good green genie out of the bottle. I now receive a growing number of e-mails from all parts of the world. Green Smoothie Challenges, in which participants commit to consuming green smoothies daily for a certain number of days or weeks, have become popular worldwide. In this photo, you can see Alaskans have to keep the lids on their smoothies so the drinks don't freeze while they are posing. Tiffany Gibson (third from left) from North Pole, Alaska, has been an avid green smoothie drinker for over two years and loves to share them with her family and friends.

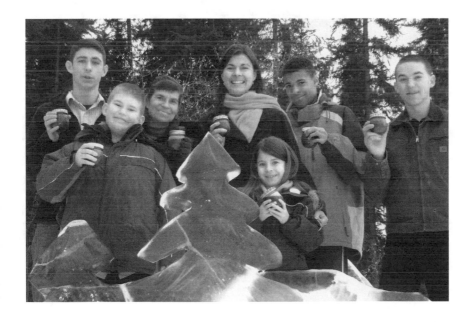

A Green Smoothie Challenge is usually organized and coordinated through the Internet, making it possible for people from distant regions to participate in the same event. For example, during the recent challenge based in Australia, more than four thousand participants from over thirty different countries drank green smoothies for two weeks. This extraordinary event was covered by a major newspaper in Australia in an article titled "Lettuce Drink to Health."[32] Anand Wells, owner of the Raw Power educational company, was the organizer of this free online health initiative. He says, "I think the green smoothie is the greatest invention of the century. It's like we have found a magic bullet." One of the supporters of the challenge in Australia, Dr. Marc Cohen, professor of complementary medicine at Melbourne's RMIT University, says, "Getting greens into the body any way you can is the important thing. I think the green smoothie is awesome. In one glass you can get more than half of your daily allowance of fruit and vegetables in one hit. If people do that, they are probably doubling or tripling the fruit and vegetable intake they otherwise would have had."[33]

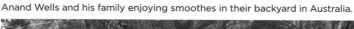

Anand Wells and his family enjoying smoothes in their backyard in Australia.

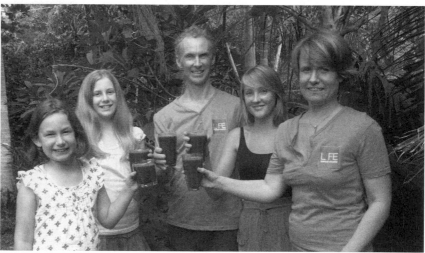

----

[32]*The Sydney Morning Herald,* November 20, 2008.
[33]Ibid.

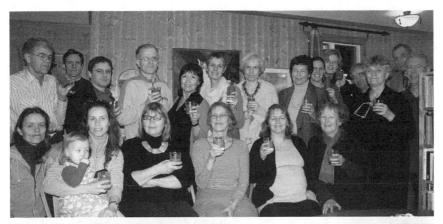

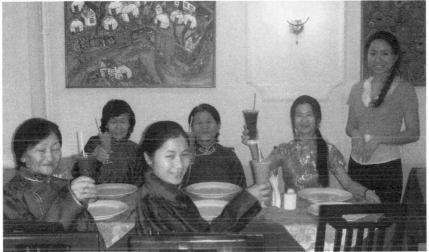

Across the world in Iceland, there are so many green smoothie drinkers that they don't even fit into the picture. Every time I travel to Iceland to teach about raw food, there are never fewer than seventy people in the audience. Sigurlina Davidsdottir (third from right, top photo) is one of the Icelandic raw food enthusiasts. She told me that long dark winters combined with the lack of locally grown produce make it difficult to stay on a raw food diet. Including green smoothies in their daily regimen has greatly helped Icelanders maintain their diet.

At Luna Blanca, a vegan and vegetarian restaurant in Mongolia, the owners now have a spinach-banana-apple smoothie on the menu.

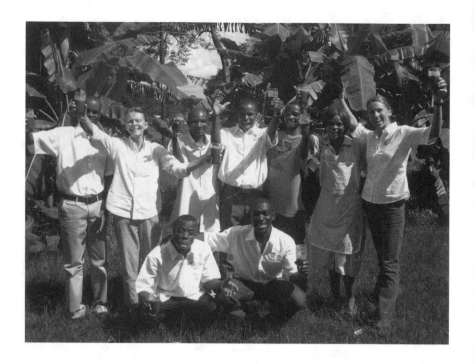

Kim Otteby (second from left) owns MyAfya, an alternative health center in Zambia, and finds green smoothies very helpful in promoting healthy living to the local population. After Kim demonstrated how to make a green smoothie on a local TV channel, many people were intrigued and started coming to the clinic. Most of her clients get to taste freshly made green smoothies at the center and want to continue drinking them. Kim found a wide variety of locally grown greens such as pumpkin leaves, rape (wild turnip), Swiss chard, sweet potato leaves, and *bondwe* (a species of amaranth). Kim says that everyone's favorite is *bondwe* for its pleasant taste. I think next I would like to travel to Zambia for some *bondwe* smoothie.

The good news about green smoothies is quickly spreading around the world. From North Pole to Africa, from Iceland to Australia, more and more people are trying this delicious drink. They quickly recognize the green smoothie miracle: a combination of simplicity, tastiness, and health benefits—and the green wave continues to spread.

APPENDIX 1
AMAZING WEIGHT LOSS: A CASE STUDY

True originality consists not in a new manner but in a new vision.
—THICH NHAT HANH

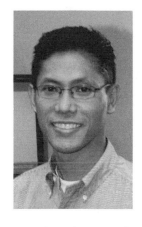

BY MIVEN DONATO, PT, DC, Health Minister, Health and Wellness Director of Dolphin Health and Education

I am a Hallelujah Acres–trained health minister. The diet and nutrition taught at Dolphin Health and Education in Medford, Oregon, is a raw food lifestyle program. While Dolphin provides chiropractic and physical therapy services that address specific clinical musculoskeletal conditions that involve diagnosis and treatment, the raw food lifestyle program does not. It is therefore prudent to check with your physician before embarking on a raw food lifestyle program. The raw food lifestyle may not be for everyone.

I have known Clent Manich since 2006. He was a patient referred to me with a diagnosis of lower back pain and sciatica. He was also a type-2 insulin-dependent diabetic and grossly obese. As a dual-licensed and practicing chiropractic physician and physical therapist, I was all too familiar with the treatment of lower back pain and sciatica. I have been a clinician since 1991 and have seen thousands of spinal cases similar to Clent's, so I expected this would be routine spinal care. But when Clent first stepped into the office, I immediately knew this was going to be a challenging case. He weighed 391 pounds at 5 feet, 11 inches tall. As a general rule, it is difficult to treat a very large person due to the limited options in spine positioning and treatment table space. Spine rehabilitation exercise is a huge challenge for grossly obese people because they are unable to get down onto the floor and get up with ease.

At the time of Clent's first office visit in late 2006, I had been introducing a lifestyle approach as adjunct to clinical work over the course of a year for treatment of chronic degenerative diseases, and back pain was one of them. In most cases a lifestyle approach to improving health is either rejected or attempted with reservation. Most patients I have encountered in the clinical setting have difficulty accepting the notion that health comes from the inside out. Patients who come to me expect that their spinal pain will be treated by spinal alignment, specific exercises, massages, or with mechanical or electrical devices.

Symptom-based treatments have been ingrained in us since childhood—when we are sick we go to the doctor for medicine. The traditional health-care mentality is deeply rooted, and Clent was no exception to this traditional thinking. What he did not know was that I wanted to try a different therapeutic approach that would not only improve his specific spine condition but also his overall health. I also wanted him to be an example, so the public would see that it is possible to overcome back pain and obesity mostly from lifestyle changes, not just chiropractic or physical therapy.

Over the years Clent had tried many popular dietary programs to help him lose weight, but he met only with disappointment. At the time of our meeting at the clinic he was well-versed enough with diet programs that he was skeptical of the raw food lifestyle. Our discussion of how health comes from the inside out, and how the body can only heal when provided with the proper building materials through wholesome raw food and lifestyle, made good sense to him. Clent was not sure he could eat mostly raw foods but was willing to give it a try. I made it clear to him that the program he was about to embark on was not just a raw diet but a lifestyle. I also made it clear to him that I would provide as much support as I could to help improve his health. In retrospect, I believe the support I provided him throughout was the key to his success in reversing diabetes and losing tremendous weight. I completely agree with Dr. Caldwell Esselstyn, MD, and his book *Prevent and Reverse Heart Disease* regarding the importance of support to prevent poor compliance to lifestyle changes.

In January 2007, Clent and his wife, Misty, signed on for the Get Healthy Boot Camp along with twenty-eight other students. There was much excitement and anticipation. The class learned how to get on the raw food lifestyle by following the Hallelujah Diet and Lifestyle founded by Reverend George Malkmus.[34] Every week I met with the class. As with other students, Clent provided me details of his weekly progress. In 7.5 weeks he lost 49.5 pounds. Clent was off his insulin medication within three weeks. His high blood pressure normalized. He was ecstatic. By boot camp graduation day at the tenth week, he reported losing a few more pounds for a total weight loss of fifty-two pounds.

Clent's confidence level was high. Following the boot camp he celebrated his overdue honeymoon with Misty by going on a cruise around the Hawaiian Islands. He told me he was very confident that he would not be tempted by food. I did not hear from him again for several months. Later, in the fall of 2007, I saw him working at Costco, pushing a grocery cart. He appeared timid when I approached him. I wanted to hear how Clent was doing. I had no intention of bringing up the subject of lifestyle, but I felt sorry for him because he did not appear well. He had gained weight since I had last seen him at boot camp graduation. He admitted he was having trouble keeping up with the lifestyle program. He was still following some of the meal schedule but also ate the wrong foods. But Clent assured me he was determined to get fully back into the program soon. I saw him again a few more times at Costco over the next several weeks. Whenever I saw him at a distance I wondered what he was going through in his personal life. I truly wanted to help this man. I saw the struggle in his face.

In early January 2008, I received a newsletter via e-mail from Victoria Boutenko that contained a link to a blog about a woman who lost 127 pounds in less than 6 months by drinking green smoothies.

---

[34]www.hacres.com

As I read the blog, I was thinking about Clent. I knew then that this information was something he needed to know. I first came across Victoria's book *Green for Life* in the latter part of 2006. My wife, Amy, came home from shopping at the Ashland Food Co-op and brought with her several of Victoria's books, including *Green for Life*. I remembered thinking that green smoothies were an excellent addition to the Hallelujah Diet meal plan and schedule I was teaching in the boot camp. I was impressed with the taste of green smoothies and their ability to satiate the appetite. As Victoria mentioned in her book, green smoothies also help curb cravings.[35] Adding the green smoothie increased the amount of raw food I could consume during the day, which gave me the boost to go higher than 85 percent raw. It could also provide the bridge necessary to go 100 percent raw.

The Hallelujah Diet and Lifestyle uses a vegan diet that is 85 percent raw foods and 15 percent cooked foods daily.[36] Unfortunately I did not fully endorse the green smoothie addition to the Hallelujah Diet during Clent's training in the 2007 boot camp until the summer. Because it was not a routine part of the meal plan, I was hesitant, but it became apparent to me that the addition of the green smoothie was a necessity to stay successful on the Hallelujah Diet. When a mutual friend, Josephine Lee, arranged a meeting between Victoria and me at the Dolphin clinic in the spring of 2007, I was overjoyed. I had questions; when I met Victoria she answered my questions and more. I realized then that Victoria's green smoothie contribution to the raw food world was enormous.

Clent responded to my e-mail saying he was very impressed with the information about the woman who lost so much weight in a short time by following Victoria's green smoothie plan. He thought if she could do it, he could do better, since he was already armed with information from the boot camp. He started drinking green smoothies in addition to the carrot juices, barley grass, and wheatgrass juices as taught in the boot camp. We discussed the fact that because of his

[35]Victoria Boutenko, *Green for Life*. (Ashland, OR: Raw Family Publishing, 2005).
[36]George Malkmus, *The Hallelujah Diet* (Shippensburg, PA: Destiny Image, 2006): 141–146.

addictions to cooked food[37] he would be better off going 100 percent raw indefinitely. I wanted Clent to beat his food problem once and for all. The first week, he lost twenty-two pounds. He was ecstatic, and I was amazed. He sent me a weekly report via e-mail and phone conversation.

Over the next several weeks he consistently averaged seven pounds of weight loss per week, or a pound a day. He was literally shrinking before my eyes. The green smoothie was the missing link to Clent's success on the Hallelujah Diet, and at 100 percent raw. I decided then that I would personally coach him through the entire weight loss ordeal until he met his goal weight of 170 pounds. Based on his consistent average weight loss per week, we calculated he would meet the target weight by Christmas 2008, in eleven months. That would be the best Christmas gift he could ever receive.

Unlike many weight loss programs that emphasize exercise along with dietary modifications, with Clent's I deferred any exercise program until he lost the first hundred pounds to prevent aggravating his lower back, which was vulnerable. After he lost 102 pounds in 14 weeks, he was ready to go to the gym. I implemented a specific exercise program that included high-intensity weight training, Dave Hubbard's Fit10 (www.fit10.com), and high-speed interval training at a high-school track. In addition, Clent also started exercising on the stair climber to train for a Mount Whitney hike. The results were amazing; Clent did not show any slowdown in his weight-loss average per week.

Clent is now nearing his anticipated goal weight of 170 pounds by December 25, 2008. His weekly average weight loss has slowed to approximately three pounds per week. At the time of this writing, October 19, 2008, Clent is at 197 pounds and has 27 pounds left to lose within nine weeks. Is this possible? We will see.

During the last nine months, Clent has gone through so many physical changes. He told me his blood work improved so much that

---

[37]Victoria Boutenko, *12 Steps to Raw Foods* (Berkeley, CA: North Atlantic Books, 2007): 87.

his primary care physician told him he no longer needed to see an endocrinologist. Clent is still free of diabetes symptoms. He is not on any prescription or over-the-counter medications and still maintains a completely raw diet. He has climbed to the summit of Mt. Whitney (14,497 feet) with Dolphin's annual Mt. Whitney hiking group. He has not only accomplished a weight loss of 204 pounds within 9 months but has also gained more than his health. As seen from his pictures posted on Dolphin's Web site, Clent has demonstrated that living a raw food lifestyle has anti-aging effects. His next plan is to write a book detailing his personal experience and to run or walk the 26.2-mile 2009 Portland marathon. His dream is to share with the world his valuable weight-loss and health-improvement experience through following the raw food lifestyle.

Clent's meal schedule is unique to his body. During the several months following a 100 percent raw diet of barley or wheatgrass juices, carrot juices, green smoothies, and raw vegetables, he encountered potentially dangerous situations with regard to his health. At his initial weight of 401 pounds on January 26, 2008, there were a lot of toxins stored in his body. At around six weeks into his diet, he experienced a major detoxification that resembled severe flu symptoms, similar to what a person fasting would experience, which Dr. Joel Fuhrman refers to as "detoxification symptoms" or "withdrawal symptoms."[38] I had to modify and delete items in Clent's daily meal plan several times and used some nutritional supplements in addition to natural methods to deal with the severe cleansing that his body went through.

While eating raw food in itself is very safe, it can bring about such a severe cleansing or detoxifying effect during the transition from cooked food that a person who does not understand these withdrawal symptoms could end up at a medical doctor's office for symptom relief or unnecessary medical intervention. Some of the unpleasant symptoms that can complicate weight loss and health improve-

---

[38]Joel Fuhrman, *Fasting and Eating for Health* (New York: St. Martin's Griffin, 1995): 18.

ment due to going on a high-raw (85 percent or more) or an all-raw diet are caused by prescription and over-the-counter medications, preexisting health challenges, and severe allergies. While not everyone will experience severe symptoms, it is important for the inexperienced raw foodist to educate himself or herself about the detoxification process and be part of a support group in the first few weeks and months of the raw food lifestyle. There are abundant resources available in bookstores and on the Internet to carefully assess whether this path is right for you. The amount of information can be overwhelming and confusing at times, so you may find it most helpful to seek out those already on a raw food diet in your community.

Clinical observation has shown me that failure to keep with the raw diet is usually due to misinterpreting the detoxification symptoms as a harmful rather than a cleansing process, and to the lack of a support system among partners, family, and friends. In my opinion, it is akin to "hitting the wall," which 26.2-mile marathon runners like me experience around the nineteenth mile. Even though Clent has gone through most of the detoxification period, it is not completely done. His weight-loss success was not easy and is not without risks. We will discuss his weight loss regime in detail in our upcoming book, hopefully to be published sometime in 2009. Educating yourself first and slowly adding raw food to your existing meal plans is the safest way to start transitioning from a Standard American Diet (SAD) to a high-raw or all-raw food lifestyle.

Clent's latest project with Victoria Boutenko is the six-week Green Smoothie Challenge (www.greensmoothierevolution.com). In response to the many questions from his Costco coworkers about his weight-loss program, Clent decided to share his dietary information with them by starting a Green Smoothie Challenge similar to the one in Australia (www.greensmoothiechallenge.com), but on a smaller scale. Due to Clent's popularity and public interest, the challenge was extended to the wider community. The kickoff was held at Lava Lanes in Medford on September 29, 2008, by Victoria Boutenko, Clent Manich, and Dr. Donato. Approximately 170 people joined in the challenge. All participants drank green smoothies daily in addition to their existing diets. The biggest "loser" received a valuable prize—a Vita-Mix blender—graciously donated by the Vita-Mix Corporation. Several other big "losers" received gifts from Costco. This green smoothie challenge brought a lot of public awareness to the possibilities of natural healing.

Dr. Donato can be reached at (541) 857-2678 at Dolphin Health and Education, 2956 E. Barnett Rd., Suite B, Medford, Oregon 97504, or www.DolphinDoctor.org.

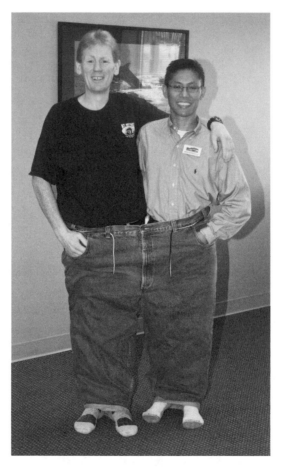

Room for two: Clent Manich and Dr. Donato in a pair of Clent's old jeans.

APPENDIX 2
CLENT MANICH: LIVING ON GREEN SMOOTHIES

Don't be afraid to give up the good to go for the great.
—KENNY ROGERS

BY CLENT MANICH

My life was difficult when I was overweight. For example, even as simple a chore as tying my own shoes seemed impossible. My wife had to tie them for me. I constantly worried about what I would do if they got untied. Getting in and out of my car was challenging because I constantly bumped into the steering wheel. Going up and down stairs was yet another demanding task. I remember that any minimal physical activity such as moving my arms left me out of breath and sweating profusely. I was weak and tired all the time.

My sleep was disturbed. I would wake up many times throughout the night. I suffered from sleep apnea, and when I woke up in the morning after eight or nine hours of sleep, I usually felt fatigued and groggy. I woke up with headaches almost every day. Consequently, I would fall asleep after meals at the dinner table. One time, my wife came into the bathroom and was surprised to find me sleeping on the toilet. I never had any energy. I attribute my fatigue partly to my restless sleep.

I wasn't accepted by many people. Some stared at me openly; others said rude things about my weight or gave me "advice" on how to lose weight. That really hurt. I brushed them all off and continued living in denial. I always desperately wanted to lose weight, but whatever I tried simply didn't work. I went on various diets countless times, only to feel weak and hungry, and eventually give up.

I was not aware of it, but I had all of the symptoms of diabetes: frequent urination, constant thirst (I would drink anything I could get my hands on), major fatigue, ears ringing all the time, a metallic taste in my mouth, and frequent dizziness.

I was scared by all these symptoms, but the worst were the heart palpitations and chest pain. I worried that my heart could stop. I kept checking the pulse on my neck to see if my heart was still beating. Eventually the chest pain became unbearable, and I checked into a hospital. I was diagnosed with acute pancreatitis. I felt as if I was having a heart attack because I had very intense pain in my chest. My blood sugar was over 600, beyond the measurement range of the glucose meter. My triglycerides were over 6,000, which meant that my bloodstream was almost entirely fat. The doctor told my wife to get the family together; he thought I might not survive. In the hospital I was given an IV and was placed on a three-day fast to get my blood-test results under control. After fasting, when I felt a little better, my doctor told me that if I didn't lose weight, I could die within three or four years. Doctors gave me an FDA-approved diet and exercise plan, which was extremely difficult to follow. I became more depressed over my condition. As a result I ate more and gained even more weight.

The turning point occurred when my weight reached four hundred pounds. At that time I tried my best to stick to the diet and exercise plan provided by my doctor. One day while exercising, I fell off a treadmill and injured myself. To treat my severe lower back pain, I was referred to Dr. Miven Donato for physical therapy. Dr. Donato told me about his Get Healthy Boot Camp, and I immediately signed up. After meeting many other people who reversed their degenerative conditions at the boot camp, I became eager to start my exercise plan. However, Dr. Donato suggested I wait until I lost a hundred pounds before starting an exercise program to avoid further injuries. I went through the boot camp and lost fifty-two pounds. Shortly after, I went on a Hawaiian cruise for my honeymoon. I thought I could handle the food, but eventually I gave in and ate what was in front of me. I gained a lot of weight back, and felt embarrassed about my failure. I avoided contact with Dr. Donato because I was ashamed of myself.

As fate would have it, I ran into Dr. Donato at Costco, where I work, and he encouraged me to get back on the program. He e-mailed me an article about a woman, Valerie, who lost 125 pounds in 25 weeks drinking green smoothies during her "Green Smoothie Experiment." I was so inspired. I decided that if she could do it, so could I. With the help and direction of Dr. Donato, I started my Green Smoothie Experiment II.

At the boot camp, we were told to drink one green smoothie a day to benefit from the great nutrition they provide. In the beginning I believed that the fruit in the smoothies was bad for my blood sugar. However, after I read the blog about Valerie's success with green smoothies, I began to understand that smoothies would nourish and heal my body. On the Internet I read many testimonials written by people who had improved their health by drinking green smoothies. I became convinced and went full-bore into drinking these nutritious mixtures every day. I also cut out animal products, fat, and dairy, and the weight started flying right off. The rapid weight loss encouraged me to stay on the diet.

Every day I drank at least four tall glasses of green smoothies. Often I started my day with a glass of carrot juice and a shot of wheat- or barley grass juice. Half an hour later I would consume sixteen ounces of green smoothie. At the beginning of each day I would blend approximately one gallon of smoothie and drink some every two to three hours. I never went longer than four hours between meals. Sometimes after drinking a green smoothie I ate a few veggies, such as pieces of carrots, celery, or cherry tomatoes. Having green smoothies for breakfast, lunch, dinner, and a later snack kept me from getting hungry. Once in a while, when I felt hungry in the evening, I would have a piece of apple, some blueberries, or other fruit. I found that smoothies helped me to eliminate food cravings better than anything I had ever tried before. By drinking smoothies every two to three hours, I stopped feeling hungry most of the time. The only thing that brought on some hunger was exercise. I believe that the high volume of fiber in green smoothies helped me to lose more weight in less time. I am still astonished that I was able to become lean and healthy, and how relatively easy it was to achieve my goals. To date I have lost 240 pounds and have attained my dream weight of 170 pounds.

I am very pleased with how my transformation has affected my relationships with other people. At work, my customers seem to be more attracted to me. My coworkers compliment me about how good I look. Of course, almost everyone asks how I did it. My friends want to make sure I'm not taking any dangerous drugs and damaging my health. Often people ask me if I had surgery. I am always delighted to spread the word about green smoothies and the Get Healthy Boot Camp.

Before my green smoothie experiment, I used to be a lot angrier. My feelings were intense, and I would often clench my jaw in anger. I was always nervous and on edge, as if expecting trouble. That feeling in my stomach, like butterflies, was a common sensation for me. I was always depressed. I cannot tell you how bad it was and how much pain my body was in. Now my attitude is more positive. I'm calmer, and I feel relaxed on a regular basis. I no longer clench my jaw. I relate to people more easily. I didn't realize the gravity of my emotional state until I started eating raw food and feeling better. I now feel confident, sane, and open in how I communicate with others.

With green smoothies, I haven't been hungry all the time like I was on other diets. Surprisingly, I consumed a lot less food on the green smoothie diet and was seldom hungry. Most other diets I've tried made me hungry and weak. That was very stressful. I never had the energy to work out, so I didn't. I always felt deprived. I had to stick to a restricted number of calories. I had to be concerned with fat and carbohydrates. I would eventually give up and go back to my old eating habits, and of course put all the weight back on. Diets never helped me in the long run. On the green smoothie experiment, I didn't have to count calories. It was very simple and easy to follow. Nobody can argue with the results: my health is the best it has ever been in my life.

After changing my diet and losing weight, my self-image also transformed. Before, I never wanted to look in the mirror; I was ashamed to even see myself. I hated the way I looked. Now I love the reflection of my body in the mirror. I say to myself, "I'm impressed! Wow. I look great!" I smile at myself. I've dreamed of this day for the last twenty years. I weigh less now than I did as a teenager. I really love my body.

The benefits I got from drinking green smoothies are numerous. For example, my gray hair changed back to my natural color; I can't find even one silver hair. The bald spot on the back of my head is gone, entirely filled in with new hair. I've grown hair on my chest and belly where I never had any before. Surprisingly, a wart disappeared from my face. One day I just noticed it was gone. My teeth have gotten whiter, and my breath sweeter. Before starting with the green smoothies, I had a sonogram on my liver. It was very enlarged then; now it is half that size. My skin is so much clearer and healthier looking. To my surprise, and to the amazement of others, unlike many other people who lose large amounts of weight, I don't have any hanging skin. My skin has tightened without any need for surgery, which I attribute entirely to the green smoothies. As you know, most people who lose this amount of weight have to spend many thousands of dollars on surgery to remove excess skin. I am grateful that my skin is so healthy. My physical strength has also increased. I am pleased with my newfound endurance, strength, and flexibility. I feel good in my body, and my thinking has gotten much clearer. Before this experiment, I was nearly blind. Recently my eye doctor asked what I'd been doing to improve my eyesight, which has become ten years younger than my age. I don't need glasses any more! I told him it was because I was drinking green smoothies every day. He said to keep it up. Now I sleep soundly through the night and only need six or seven hours to feel refreshed upon waking. I get up at 5 a.m. to exercise at the gym before going to work. I have been drinking smoothies for a year, since January 26, 2008, and I haven't missed a day yet!

In addition to my regular job, I have become a teacher and nutritional speaker. I teach a couple of classes at the community college, helping others learn how to lose weight the way I did. I give monthly talks in my community, sharing the story of how green smoothies and the raw diet have changed my health and my life. I have so much compassion for others who are still suffering and try to encourage them to get better.

I am creating a Web site, www.clentmanich.com, to tell my story and keep people up-to-date on my progress. The site will have a blog where I answer the thousands of questions I receive about how I regained my health. I will also post answers to the most frequently asked questions. I enjoy teaching people about what I've done. One day, I may even be able to do it full-time. Getting healthy has opened a lot of new doors for me.

I am dedicated to drinking green smoothies for the rest of my life. For the past year, they have been the main course in my diet. Since I have reached my goal weight of 170 pounds, I have gradually added some more raw dishes. But I continue drinking at least one green smoothie a day. By now my smoothies have become supergreen. Sometimes I combine two bunches of greens into one smoothie. My next goal is to prove that I can keep this weight off for five years.

The following is a detailed description of my daily diet:

In the morning I usually drink a twelve-ounce fresh carrot juice mixed with wheatgrass juice. Next I prepare about a gallon of green smoothie, enough to supply four meals throughout the day. I usually add half an avocado and two tablespoons of ground flaxseed to my daily smoothie. I consume my green smoothies throughout the day, a large cup every two to three hours, until I finish it. Along with the smoothie meals, during the day I snack on a wide variety of raw veggies such as celery sticks, baby carrots, asparagus, sweet peppers, zucchini, or broccoli. Every day my snacks are different, but I always drink a smoothie. Once in a while, when I crave something sweet, I grab a banana, or a peach, or a handful of grape tomatoes, but in

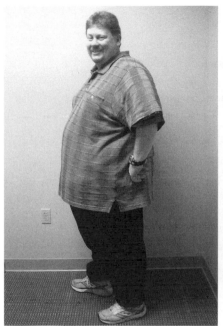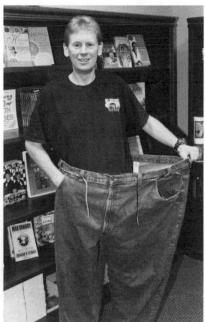

First photo: January 26, 2008, when I weighed 400.6 pounds.
Second photo: January 20, 2009, at 170 pounds.

general I consume fruit in moderation. I do not add any nuts, seeds, salt, or oils. I drink lots of water all day long. This way I have enough to eat in a day to control my hunger.

In the very beginning of my experiment I weighed over four hundred pounds, and I was hurting myself during exercise. Dr. Donato asked me to wait until I was under three hundred pounds to start exercising. I lost 102 pounds in fourteen weeks without exercising. Now I train with weights three times a week at the local gym under the supervision of Dr. Donato, along with light cardio-anaerobic exercise daily.

CLENT'S WEIGHT-LOSS PROGRESS LOG

1/26/08:	400.6 lbs.		Today I began "The Green Smoothie Experiment II."
2/23/08:	356.0	(-7.0)	My coworkers notice my face looks thinner 2/21
2/16/08:	363.0	(-7.6)	Hard-core cold symptoms on 2/12
2/09/08:	370.6	(-7.4)	Down one pant size on 2/08

2/02/08:	378.0	(-22.6)	Wow! What a start!
3/15/08:	337.6	(-6.6)	Major flu symptoms on 3/10
3/08/08:	344.2	(-4.8)	Started food enzymes to protect my liver on 3/02
3/01/08:	349.0	(-7.0)	Down two pant sizes on 2/28
3/22/08:	330.6	(-7.0)	Down three pant sizes on 3/16
3/29/08:	325.4	(-5.2)	Sleeping less (about 6–7 hours per night) and feeling better
4/05/08:	320.0	(-5.4)	Less pain in my feet and lower back after 8 hours at work
4/12/08:	314.8	(-5.2)	Eyesight has reversed to 10 years younger than my age
4/19/08:	309.6	(-5.2)	Liver has improved, and fat deposits in liver have reduced
4/26/08:	304.6	(-5.0)	Able to bend over, cross my legs, and tie my shoes without effort
5/03/08:	298.2	(-6.4)	Down four pant sizes on 5/01. Under 300 lbs. on 5/02
5/10/08:	293.6	(-4.6)	Began phase 2 cardio and weight training with Dr. Donato on 5/04
5/17/08:	289.6	(-4.0)	Coworkers let me know they are amazed at my weight loss
5/24/08:	283.8	(-5.8)	Down five pant sizes and at weight-loss halfway mark on 5/20
5/31/08:	278.6	(-5.2)	Down six pant sizes on 05/28. Began anaerobic exercise
6/07/08:	273.4	(-5.2)	I passed Valerie's 127-lb. loss 7 weeks sooner, on 6/06
6/14/08:	268.0	(-5.4)	Down seven pant sizes (56 to 42), and 14 inches off waist on 6/13
6/21/08:	265.0	(-3.0)	It's official: I no longer have diabetes!
6/28/08:	258.6	(-6.4)	My skin is shrinking nicely, as expected on a raw diet!
7/05/08:	254.6	(-4.0)	In parade with Boutenko family and friends on Fourth of July (their float won first place!)
7/12/08:	249.6	(-5.0)	Able to fit into a 2X shirt, down from 5X on 7/10
7/19/08:	245.2	(-4.4)	On 7/16 I began training for the hike up Mt. Whitney
7/26/08:	240.0	(-5.2)	Down eight pant sizes on 7/21. Six months 100% raw!

Total lost by 8/02/08: 164 lbs., 100-percent raw!

Mount Whitney is the highest summit in the contiguous United States, with an elevation of 14,505 feet. I joined Dr. Donato and friends on September 2, 2008 to climb Mount Whitney, and made it to the summit!

HOW THE RAW FAMILY WENT RAW

We joke in my family that we were fortunate to get sick all together, but back then, in 1993, our health problems were no joke. All four of us (my husband, our two children, and myself) were deathly sick. Our family of five had emigrated from Russia in 1989 when I was invited by Denver Community College to teach about perestroika. At that time in Russia there was a shortage of food, and our diet was limited to what was available, which was mostly grains, dairy products, and some fruit. When we came to America, we were amazed at the variety and availability of food, and we started trying everything. We loved the convenience of prepackaged food. I remember that we enjoyed using a microwave often. Within three years, four of us were diagnosed with deadly diseases that included arrhythmia and edema (Victoria), hyperthyroidism and rheumatoid arthritis (Igor), allergies and asthma (Valya), and diabetes (Sergei). Our oldest son Stephan was the only one in our family who escaped severe illness.

When the doctors told us that our conditions were incurable, we did not want to believe them, and started looking for an alternative way of healing. My search was intense; for several months I couldn't do anything but go around asking people about health. I read nonstop in libraries, attended lectures and seminars, and met with various health practitioners.

Eventually I ran into Elizabeth, a woman who was probably one of the only raw foodists at that time in Colorado. She was the first person I met who felt confident that our illnesses could be reversed. Elizabeth told me she had cured her stage-four colon cancer twenty years earlier through eating raw food. At first, I was disappointed. I was looking for a more serious solution. I was willing to work hard and pay any amount of money for some miraculous herb or treatment. Raw food sounded absurd to me—too simplistic. I'd heard of raw foods before, but I was not so naïve to believe in that kind of diet. So I asked Elizabeth, "Do you really believe that humans can survive on just fruits, vegetables, nuts, and seeds, raw?!"

Elizabeth responded with three indisputable arguments: (1) animals do not cook; (2) she had been eating only raw food for twenty years and healed her colon cancer; (3) we did not come into this world with a cooking stove attached to our belly. These points were far from scientific, but I couldn't think of anything to refute them. Besides, I was greatly impressed with Elizabeth's youthful look, and I desperately wanted everyone in my family to feel better. Elizabeth loaned me a book about raw food and gave me her phone number. I went home and started reading.

Bear in mind that in 1993 there were only a few books about raw food available and they were not sold in stores, only from the authors themselves. I quickly read the book that Elizabeth loaned me and suddenly the promise of the raw food diet seemed so obvious. Next, though, I became scared. I thought, "Now I have to give up the last pleasure I have left in life." At the same time, I was already eager to try raw food and see if it would work for my family. Igor and I agreed to try a raw food diet for two weeks, to see if there would be any improvement in our health at all.

In the morning of January 21st, 1994 I went into the kitchen. I fully realized that this could be the only chance in a lifetime to make such a drastic change. Therefore, I was decisive. I carefully examined the food that we had in the fridge and in the cupboards and discovered that we had almost zero raw food in our house. Everything had to go! I took a heavy-duty garbage bag and cleaned out all the beans, macaroni, cereal, rice, TV dinners, popsicles, whipped cream, breads, sauces, cheese, and cans of tuna. Next went the coffeemaker, toaster, and pasta maker. I turned off the pilot light and covered the stove with a large cutting board. Now our kitchen looked as if we were moving out. The only item left on the counter was our huge, expensive micro-wave oven. When we lived in Russia, we couldn't have one because Russian scientists performed research and found out that microwave ovens were very harmful. For this reason microwave ovens were pro-hibited in Russia. As a result, when we came to the United States, we bought a big one. Now I was staring at this microwave oven and real-ized that I didn't know what to do about it. I started thinking about delicious melted cheese sandwiches, Pop Tarts, and all the "miracles" I used to bake in it. Then I thought about Sergei and his diabetes. Most of all in the world, I did not want him to go on insulin. So I got a hammer and cracked the microwave's glass door, then put it in the garage. I put all our brand-new pots and pans that I'd just gotten for Christmas out on the sidewalk, and they disappeared minutes later. Then I rushed to the local supermarket.

At that time I was not aware of the existence of raw gourmet dishes. I didn't know what raw fooders ate, having never met any besides Elizabeth, who ate simply. I had never heard of dehydrated flax crackers, nut milks, seed cheese, or raw cakes. I thought of raw food as mainly being salads. Furthermore, I came from Russia, where fresh fruits and vegetables were available only during the summer. We were used to eating potatoes, meat, macaroni, lots of dairy prod-ucts, and occasionally fruit. We were not accustomed to eating sal-ads, and my family didn't like vegetables. Therefore, I was confined to the fruit section of the produce department. Due to our tight bud-get, we usually bought only Washington apples, naval oranges, and bananas. I loaded my cart with these three items.

When my kids came home from school and Igor from work, they asked, "What's for dinner?" I told them to look in the fridge. My chil-dren couldn't believe their eyes. "Where are our TV dinners? Where did all the ice cream go?" They threw a fit. Sergei said, "I would rather take insulin shots for the rest of my life than stay on such a crazy diet." They refused to eat and went to their rooms to watch videos.

Igor ate a couple of bananas and complained that this food made him hungrier. We had lots of time that day. I remember everyone walking from one room to another looking at the clock. This was my initial realization of how much of my time had been spent thinking about, planning, preparing to eat, eating, and cleaning up afterwards. We felt hungry, uncomfortable, weird, and lost. We tried watching TV, but the grilled chicken commercials were unbearable. We hardly made it to nine o'clock. Unable to fall asleep due to my own empty stomach, I heard footsteps in our kitchen and the sound of cupboards opening and closing.

In the morning, we woke up unusually early and gathered in the kitchen. I noticed lots of peels from bananas and oranges on the counter. Valya shared with us that she hadn't coughed that night. I remember telling her, "That is just a coincidence; the diet couldn't work that fast." Sergei checked his blood sugar. It was still high, but *it was lower* than it had been for several weeks. Igor and I noticed a slight energy increase, and generally felt lighter and more positive. We were also very hungry.

I have never told anyone that shifting to a raw food diet was easy. In fact, it was very hard for the four of us. Our bodies were demanding the foods we used to eat. From the very first day, and for a couple weeks, minute after minute, I was daydreaming of eating bagels with cream cheese, hot soups, chocolate, or, at the very least, various types of chips. At night in my sleep, I was searching for French fries under my pillow. I snuck two dollars from the family piggy bank and kept them in my pocket. I kept plotting that one day I would have half an hour alone to run down to the corner restaurant and buy a slice of hot, cheesy pizza, eat it fast without being seen, run back, and continue the raw food diet. Luckily, I never found that chance.

At the very same time, positive changes rapidly appeared. Valya stopped coughing at night and never had an asthmatic attack again. Sergei's blood sugar steadily began to stabilize. Igor's swelling in his throat subsided to normal. His pulse went down, and the symptoms of hyperthyroidism became less apparent with each day. I noticed that my clothes were loose on my body, even when they were fresh out of the dryer. That had never happened before. I was excited! Every morning, I ran to the mirror and examined my face, counting the disappearing wrinkles. My face definitely looked better and younger with each day of the raw life.

After one month on raw food, Sergei asked me why he had to check his blood sugar every three hours when it was now consistently within the normal range. I told him to check it only once, in the morning. Valya was able to run a quarter of a mile at school without coughing. Igor's pulse normalized, and I lost fifteen pounds. All of us noticed that we had a lot more energy. We decided to start running as a family. Eventually, Sergei's blood sugar stabilized due to his new diet and regular jogging. From the day that we began to eat raw food to the present, he has never again experienced any form of diabetic symptoms.

We appreciated that our health was quickly restored to normal and that we had become even healthier than ever before. To share the story of our amazing healing with as many people as possible, and to inspire others to try this dietary approach, we published a book about our experiences called *Raw Family: A True Story of Awakening.*

WHAT WAS MISSING IN OUR RAW FOOD PLAN?

After several years of being raw-foodists, each one of us began to feel like we had reached a plateau where our healing processes had stopped, and had even begun to go backwards. About seven years into our completely raw diet, more and more often we started feeling discontent with our existing food program. I began to have a heavy feeling in my stomach after eating almost any kind of raw food, especially a salad with dressing. Because of that, I started to eat fewer greens and more fruits and nuts. I began to gain weight. My husband started to develop a lot of gray hair.

My family members felt confused about our diet and started asking more often "What should we eat?" There were times when we felt hungry but did not desire any foods that were "legal" for us to eat on our diet of vegetables, fruits, nuts, seeds, grains, sprouts, and dried fruit. Salads with dressings were delicious but made us tired and sleepy. We felt trapped. I remember Igor looking inside the fridge, saying over and over again, "I wish I wanted some of this stuff."

These periods did not last. We blamed it all on stress and overeating and were able to refresh our appetites by fasts, exercise, hikes, or by working more. In my family we strongly believe that raw food is the only way to go so we encouraged each other to maintain our raw diet no matter what, always trying new variations with our food. Many of my friends told me about similar experiences, at which point they gave up being 100 percent raw and began to add cooked food back into their meals. In my family, we continued to stay on raw food due to our constant support of each other.

But a burning question began to grow stronger in my heart with each day. The question was, "Is there anything missing in our diet?" The answer would come right away: "Nope. Nothing could be better than a raw food diet. This diet saved our lives." Still, the unwanted signs of less-than-perfect health kept surfacing in minor but noticeable symptoms, such as a wart on a hand or a gray hair, symptoms that brought doubts about the completeness of the raw food diet. Finally, when my children complained about the increased sensitivity of their teeth, I reached a state where I couldn't think about anything besides this health puzzle. I drove everybody around me crazy with my constant discussion of what could possibly be missing.

Due to lack of information in those early years, we made a lot of mistakes. For example, we consumed too many nuts, seeds, and oils. The bulk of our diet consisted of root vegetables and fruit. For the first couple years we were eating conventionally grown produce, as we did not appreciate organic food. Our biggest oversight, it turns out, was that we consumed very few greens.

I started conducting a lot of research and in 2004 I came to the conclusion that the missing ingredient in our diet was green leaves. After incorporating plenty of greens into our diets in the form of green smoothies, all of our minor health problems completely vanished. Finally, we felt vibrant.

Ever since I first described our story in my books, readers have asked me, "So, does the raw food diet work?" After more than fifteen years of practicing the raw food diet, I consider the optimal diet for humans to be as much raw food as possible, with a huge emphasis on greens. Still, many people ask, "What is more important: to be 100 percent raw, or to consume large amounts of greens regularly?" I gave this tough question a lot of thought and research, and my conclusion is that eating enough greens is definitely more important. Those who can combine greens with an all-raw diet will reap the most health benefits. However, I've had plenty of opportunity to observe how difficult this goal is for many people. Therefore, the best way to start is by enjoying green smoothies!

INDEX

Alfalfa sprouts
 Sweet Tart Smoothie, 104
Alkaloids, 19–20, 48
All Kinds of Peppers and Tomatoes,
 84
Aloe vera
 Aloe Facial Cleanser, 129
 "Bitter Delight" Cocktail, 98
 Green Smoothie Monster, 73
 Green Star, 103
 Green Stinger, 78
 The Pear-fect Smoothie, 107
 Rocket Fuel Smoothie, 60
 Sunlight on Soil, 114
 Today's Discovery, 104
Andrea's Green Delight, 68
Animals, green smoothies for, 41–44,
 127–28
Anticancer Smoothie, 75
Antioxidant Longevity Smoothie, 105
Antioxidants, 25, 28–29
Aphrodisiacs
 Aphrodisiac Cocktail, 100
 O-Mega Aphrodisiac, 97
Apple juice
 Bleh! "So Bland, Why Did I Try
  This, But It's Growing on Me"
  Smoothie, 99
 Dancing Dandelion Smoothie, 58
 Dandy Lions, 74
 Dent de Lion, 58
 Frozen Mango Mint, 120
 Gooseberry Crush, 62
 Heavy Metals Be Gone, 77
 World's Safest Liver Cleanser, 78

Apples
 Andrea's Green Delight, 68
 Apple Green Smoothie, 64
 Applesauce, 108
 Blue Skies Green Smoothie, 67
 Bok Choy Joy, 88
 Citrus Sunlight, 70
 Coconut Dream Pudding, 116
 Colon Surprise Pudding, 113
 Emerald Applesauce, 121
 Favorite Green Smoothie, 66
 Fido's Dream, 128
 Good Stuff, 68
 Green Smoothie with Miner's
  Lettuce, 106
 I Can't Believe It's Green Smoothie,
  67
 Lovely Green Goodness, 62
 Memory Booster Brain Smoothie,
  61
 Parsley Passion Smoothie, 58
 Pineapple Pudding Waltz, 117
 Pink and Green, 61
 Prickly Anticancer Recipe, 75
 Prickly Pear Green-Go, 101
 Recette des Champs Congelés, 116
 Red Smoothie, 71
 Revolution-Evolution, 66
 Sea Buckthorn Rumba, 99
 Spinach Pudding, 117
 Splendid Calendula, 110
 Springtime Douglas Fir Smoothie,
  105
 Summertime Smoothie, 71
 Sweet Parsley Smoothie, 62

Apples, *continued*
  Sweet Soup, 95
  Valya's Green Pudding, 112
Apricots
  Apricot Nectar, 122
  Silly Cilantro, 102
  Summer Splendor Smoothie, 97
Arugula
  Coconut Chameleon, 115
  Morning Spark, 102
  Orange Aid, 93
  Orange Zest, 94
Avocados
  All Kinds of Peppers and Tomatoes, 84
  Aloe Facial Cleanser, 129
  Avo-Coco Pudding, 111
  Banacado, 114
  Celery Soup, 94
  Coco-nash Smoothie, 125
  Cool Summer Smoothie, 86
  Cucumber Dill-icious Soup, 82
  Fennel Soup, 87
  Garden Walk, 85
  Herb Garden, 90
  Hot Stuff, 106
  Immune Booster, 91
  Mediterranean Soup, 81
  Mustard Musketeer, 84
  Neighbor's Garden, 83
  Oregano Tummy Soother, 82
  Original Raw Family Smoothie Improved, 61
  Papayavocado Pudding, 109
  Probiotic Guacamole Spread, 93
  Raw Family Green Soup, 95
  Savory Basil Soup, 85
  Savory Cucumber Lassi, 87
  Scarlet Honey Mustard Spread, 93
  Soup Gazpacho, 82
  Spicy Green Soup, 86
  Sweet Soup, 95
  Thai Soup, 83
Avocado seeds, 54
  Bleh! "So Bland, Why Did I Try This, But It's Growing on Me" Smoothie, 99

Baby greens
  All Kinds of Peppers and Tomatoes, 84

Pineapple Pudding Waltz, 117
Banacado, 114
Bananas
  Andrea's Green Delight, 68
  Applesauce, 108
  Apricot Nectar, 122
  Avo-Coco Pudding, 111
  Banacado, 114
  "Bitter Delight" Cocktail, 98
  Bleh! "So Bland, Why Did I Try This, But It's Growing on Me" Smoothie, 99
  For the Brave, 76
  Citrus Sunlight, 70
  Clementine Citrus Circus, 123
  Coconut Chameleon, 115
  Coconut Dream Pudding, 116
  Colon Surprise Pudding, 113
  Daily Meal, 79
  Dreamsicle Smoothie, 115
  Durian Green Pudding, 111
  Every Morning, 67
  Favorite Green Smoothie, 66
  Good Stuff, 68
  Grandiose Grape Smoothie, 121
  Greena Colada, 63
  Green Jungle Jamboree, 76
  Green Smoothie Monster, 73
  Green Smoothie Popsicles!, 125
  Green Strawberry Drink, 125
  Kent Mango Bliss, 108
  The Laughing Gorilla, 119
  Lemon Pudding, 111
  Lovely Green Goodness, 62
  Mango-Lime Pudding, 109
  Morning Spark, 102
  Oh Bay-Beh Bay-Beh, 100
  One Tough Banana, 89
  Orange Zest, 94
  Original Raw Family Smoothie Improved, 61
  Parsley Passion Smoothie, 58
  The Pear-fect Smoothie, 107
  Persimmon Pudding, 107
  Pineapple Spice Cake, 70
  Poochie's Gourmet Green Smoothie, 127
  P-P-Papaya Smoothie, 59
  Prickly Pear Green-Go, 101
  Purple Teeth Masquerade, 123
  Red Bandit, 110

Saskatoon Sunrise, 65
Sea Buckthorn Rumba, 99
Shelah's Tangy Pudding, 109
Spinach Freshness, 124
Spinach Pudding, 117
Springtime Douglas Fir Smoothie, 105
Steven's Tropical Wigmore-Inspired Energy Smoothie, 105
Summertime Smoothie, 71
Sun Green Pudding, 114
Sweet and Salty Star Pudding, 113
Sweet and Sour, 124
Sweet Parsley Smoothie, 62
Sweet Tart Smoothie, 104
Three-Course Meal, 115
Thunderstorm Smoothie, 60
Today's Discovery, 104
Tropical Green Smoothie, 65
Wheat Grass-Hopper, 72
Wicked Watermelon Smoothie, 59
World's Safest Liver Cleanser, 78
Basic Balance, 57
Basil
    Celery Zing Soup, 94
    Herb Garden, 90
    Jim's Basic Basil, 87
    Savory Basil Soup, 85
    Soup Gazpacho, 82
    Spicy Green Soup, 86
Beet greens
    For the Brave, 76
    Grandiose Grape Smoothie, 121
    Red Bandit, 110
    Red Smoothie, 71
    Scarlet Honey Mustard Spread, 93
    Summertime Smoothie, 71
Beets
    Scarlet Honey Mustard Spread, 93
Bell peppers
    All Kinds of Peppers and Tomatoes, 84
    Celery Zing Soup, 94
    Hot Stuff, 106
    Mediterranean Soup, 81
    Orange Aid, 93
    Orange Zest, 94
    Satisfying Smoothie, 79
    Savory Basil Soup, 85
    Soup Gazpacho, 82
    Spicy Green Soup, 86

Berries. *See also individual berries*
    Berry Blue Smoothie, 120
    Green Smoothie Popsicles!, 125
    Recette des Champs Congelés, 116
    Winter Green Smoothie, 63, 72
"Bitter Delight" Cocktail, 98
Blackberries
    Anticancer Smoothie, 75
    Berry Blue Smoothie, 120
    Purple Teeth Masquerade, 123
    Yummerific, 66
Black Sheep, 68
Bleh! "So Bland, Why Did I Try This, But It's Growing on Me" Smoothie, 99
Blenders, 53
Blending
    juicing vs., 27–30
    time for, 53
Bloody Mary, 106
Blueberries
    Berry Blue Smoothie, 120
    Black Sheep, 68
    Blueberry Zing, 109
    Blue Skies Green Smoothie, 67
    Double Green Smoothie, 74
    Dreamsicle Smoothie, 115
    Every Morning, 67
    Lambsquarters Omega Pudding, 112
    Miner's Lettuce Smoothie, 120
    Purple Green Smoothie, 95
    Saskatoon Sunrise, 65
    Simply Delicious Double-Green Pudding, 80
Blue Skies Green Smoothie, 67
Body care, green smoothies for, 129
Bok choy
    Bok Choy Joy, 88
    For the Brave, 76
    Dilly Crazy Baby Bok Choy, 91
    Mustard Musketeer, 84
    Tooty Fruity, 100
Borage
    Oh Bay-Beh Bay-Beh, 100
Boutenko, Sergei and Valya, 54
Broccoli
    Anticancer Smoothie, 75
Buckwheat sprouts
    Bleh! "So Bland, Why Did I Try This, But It's Growing on Me" Smoothie, 99

Butter lettuce
European Black Currant Smoothie, 60
Goji Berry Enchantment, 63
Perfectly Peachy, 59

Cactus
Cactus Green Smoothie, 80
Prickly Pear Green-Go, 101
Calcium, 34
Calendula flowers and leaves
Mustard Musketeer, 84
Splendid Calendula, 110
Cancer, 10–11, 13, 30, 75
Cantaloupe
Cantaloupe Parsley Smoothie, 57
Medallion Melon Smoothie, 59
Wild Melon Smoothie, 100
Carrots
Mustard Musketeer, 84
Carrot tops
For the Brave, 76
Neighbor's Garden, 83
Rabbit Patch, 92
Cashews
Strawberry Crème, 112
Cats, green smoothies for, 41–44, 128
Celery
Avo-Coco Pudding, 111
Bloody Mary, 106
Bok Choy Joy, 88
Celery Soup, 94
Celery Zing Soup, 94
Cucumber Dill-icious Soup, 82
Dreamsicle Smoothie, 115
Fennel Soup, 87
Goji Berry Enchantment, 63
Green Strawberry Drink, 125
Heavy Metals Be Gone, 77
Hot Stuff, 106
I Can't Believe It's Green Smoothie, 67
Jim's Basic Basil, 87
Liver Lover, 88
Mediterranean Soup, 81
Morning Zing Smoothie, 57
Radical Radish, 90
Raw Family Green Soup, 95
Savory Cucumber Lassi, 87
Sea Buckthorn Rumba, 99

Shelah's Tangy Pudding, 109
Soup Gazpacho, 82
Spicy Sinus Cleaner, 77
Summer Splendor Smoothie, 97
Sweet Soup, 95
Today's Discovery, 104
Chard
"Bitter Delight" Cocktail, 98
Coconut Dream Pudding, 116
Green Smoothie Monster, 73
Green Star, 103
I Can't Believe It's Green Smoothie, 67
Kent Mango Bliss, 108
Mango-Lime Pudding, 109
Mango Tarragon, 92
Pineapple Spice Cake, 70
Prickly Pear Green-Go, 101
Raw Family Green Soup, 95
Satisfying Smoothie, 79
Steven's Tropical Wigmore-Inspired Energy Smoothie, 105
Summer Splendor Smoothie, 97
Sweet and Salty Star Pudding, 113
Thunderstorm Smoothie, 60
Valya's Green Pudding, 112
Chavez, Gabrielle, 21
Chicken Scratch, 78
Chickweed
"Bitter Delight" Cocktail, 98
Chicken Scratch, 78
Green Jungle Jamboree, 76
Children, green smoothies for, 37–39, 119–26
Chili peppers
Garden Walk, 85
Hot Stuff, 106
Mediterranean Soup, 81
Morning Glory, 89
Orange Aid, 93
Spicy Sinus Cleaner, 77
Chimpanzees, diet of, 15–16, 17–18
Chlorophyll, 3
Christmas in June, 69
Cilantro
All Kinds of Peppers and Tomatoes, 84
Avo-Coco Pudding, 111
Bok Choy Joy, 88
Cilantro Sparkle, 113

Heavy Metals Be Gone, 77
Morning Glory, 89
Red Smoothie, 71
Silly Cilantro, 102
Sunlight on Soil, 114
Citrus Sunlight, 70
Clementine Citrus Circus, 123
Coconuts
Avo-Coco Pudding, 111
choosing, 54
Coco-nash Smoothie, 125
Coconut Chameleon, 115
Coconut Dream Pudding, 116
Coco-Tango, 119
Dreamsicle Smoothie, 115
Greena Colada, 63
Green Monkey Face, 124
Hawaiian Hibiscus, 101
Lambsquarters Omega Pudding,
112
opening, 54–55
removing meat from, 56
Strawberry Crème, 112
Cohen, Marc, 132
Cold Buster, Spinach, 92
Collard greens
Green Caprice, 103
Sweet Tart Smoothie, 104
Colon Surprise Pudding, 113
Constipation, 36
Cool Summer Smoothie, 86
Cranberries
Blue Skies Green Smoothie, 67
Red Bandit, 110
World's Safest Liver Cleanser, 78
Cucumbers
Aloe Facial Cleanser, 129
Cool Summer Smoothie, 86
Cucumber Dill-icious Soup, 82
Dark Green Love, 74
Herb Garden, 90
Immune Booster, 91
Mediterranean Soup, 81
Memory Booster Brain Smoothie,
61
Mustard Musketeer, 84
Oregano Tummy Soother, 82
Parsley Passion Smoothie, 58
Purple Green Smoothie, 95
Rabbit Patch, 92

Refreshing Cucumber Spinach, 91
Savory Cucumber Lassi, 87
Spicy Sinus Cleaner, 77
Spinach Cold Buster, 92
Thai Soup, 83
Curly kale
Clementine Citrus Circus, 123
Thai Soup, 83
Currant Smoothie, European Black,
60

Daily Meal, 79
Dancing Dandelion Smoothie, 58
Dandelion greens
Blue Skies Green Smoothie, 67
Coconut Chameleon, 115
Dancing Dandelion Smoothie, 58
Dandy Lions, 74
Dark Green Love, 74
Dent de Lion, 58
Double Green Smoothie, 74
Forest Full of Trees, 98
Green Smoothie Monster, 73
Honeydew & Dandelion, 99
Liver Lover, 88
Morning Zing Smoothie, 57
Saskatoon Sunrise, 65
Simply Delicious Double-Green
Pudding, 80
Velvet Green Smoothie, 80
Victoria's Favorite Dark Green, 73
World's Safest Liver Cleanser, 78
Yummerific, 66
Dandy Lions, 74
Dark Green Love, 74
Dates
Apple Green Smoothie, 64
Banacado, 114
Coconut Dream Pudding, 116
Delicious Spring Green Smoothie,
126
Red Bandit, 110
Sun Green Pudding, 114
Sweet and Sour, 124
Sweet Parsley Smoothie, 62
Sweet Tart Smoothie, 104
Three-Course Meal, 115
Davidsdottir, Sigurlina, 133
Delicious Spring Green Smoothie, 126
Dent de Lion, 58

Dentist's Nightmare Smoothie, 123
Detoxification, 140–41
Dill
  Cool Summer Smoothie, 86
  Cucumber Dill-icious Soup, 82
  Dilly Crazy Baby Bok Choy, 91
  Neighbor's Garden, 83
  Probiotic Guacamole Spread, 93
  Sweet Soup, 95
Dinosaur kale, 19
  Celery Zing Soup, 94
  Cucumber Dill-icious Soup, 82
  Original Raw Family Smoothie
    Improved, 61
  Purple Teeth Masquerade, 123
  Revitalizing Energizer Smoothie, 98
  Revolution-Evolution, 66
  Shelah's Tangy Pudding, 109
Dogs, green smoothies for, 41–44, 127
Dolphin Health and Education, 135,
  138, 140, 142
Donaldson, Michael, 29
Donato, Miven, 135–42, 144–45,
  149–50
Double Green Pudding, 117
Double Green Smoothie, 74
Douglas Fir Smoothie, Springtime,
  105
Dreamsicle Smoothie, 115
Drewnowski, Adam, 25
Dulse
  Mustard Musketeer, 84
  Savory Basil Soup, 85
Durian Green Pudding, 111

Emerald Applesauce, 121
Endive
  World's Safest Liver Cleanser, 78
Esselstyn, Caldwell, 136
European Black Currant Smoothie, 60
Every Morning, 67

Facial Cleanser, Aloe, 129
Fats, 36
Favorite Green Smoothie, 66
Fennel
  Fennel Soup, 87
  Herb Garden, 90
  Radical Radish, 90
  What a Pair!, 89

Fiber, 30, 36, 46, 54
Fido's Dream, 128
Figs
  Black Sheep, 68
  Fig Fantasy, 70
  Turkish Grove, 69
Fluffy's Delight, 128
Food combining, 45–46
Forest Full of Trees, 98
For the Brave, 76
Frisée lettuce
  Bleh! "So Bland, Why Did I Try
    This, But It's Growing on Me"
    Smoothie, 99
Frozen Mango Mint, 120
Fruits. See also individual fruits
  blending, 53–54
  in chimpanzee diet, 16, 17
  green, 45–46
  organic, 48–49
  peeling, 53–54
  recommended, 54
  rotating, 20, 48
  sweet, 33
Fruity Weeds, 104
Fuhrman, Joel, 140

Garden Walk, 85
Garlic
  Spinach Cold Buster, 92
Gazpacho, Soup, 82
Gerson, Max, 11
Get Healthy Boot Camp, 137, 144,
  146
Gibson, Tiffany, 131
Goji berries and leaves
  Goji Berry Enchantment, 63
  Sea Buckthorn Rumba, 99
Goodall, Jane, 17
Good Stuff, 68
Gooseberry Crush, 62
Graham, Doug, 30
Grandiose Grape Smoothie, 121
Grapefruit
  Midsummer, 75
  Peachy Keen Green, 102
Grape leaves
  Green Pudding, 108
  Resveratrol Elixir of Life, 76
  Revitalizing Energizer Smoothie, 98

Grapes
  Bleh! "So Bland, Why Did I Try
    This, But It's Growing on Me"
    Smoothie, 99
  Cactus Green Smoothie, 80
  Grandiose Grape Smoothie, 121
  Green Stinger, 78
  Prickly Anticancer Recipe, 75
  Purple Green Smoothie, 95
  Rocket Fuel Smoothie, 60
Greena Colada, 63
Green Caprice, 103
Green Julius, 69
Green Jungle Jamboree, 76
Green Monkey Face, 124
Green Pudding, 108
Greens. *See also individual greens*
  abundance of, 7
  alkaloids in, 19–20, 48
  bitter, 24–25
  in chimpanzee diet, 16, 17
  cultivated, 21
  daily consumption of, 31
  definition of, 45
  dried, 34
  frozen, 33
  harvesting, 5
  in history, 7–8
  incorporating, into diet, 15, 17–18
  list of, 21–22
  measuring, 56
  nutrition and, 5, 7–8, 13–14, 25
  organic, 48–49
  rotating, 19–20, 25, 48
  stalks of, 54
  wild, 22, 24, 35
Green Smoothie Challenges, 131–32,
  141
Green Smoothie Monster, 73
Green Smoothie Popsicles!, 125
Green smoothies. *See also individual*
    recipes
  advantages of, 30
  for adventurous souls, 97–106
  for beginners, 57–72
  for body care, 129
  for children, 37–39, 119–26
  daily consumption of, 33
  dried greens in, 34
  fat in, 36

food combining in, 45–46
frothiness of, 54
guidelines for, 47–49
origin of, 17–18
for pets, 41–44, 127–28
preparing, 53–56
revolution of, 131–34
rotating greens in, 19–20, 25, 48
storing, 33–34
supergreen, 73–80
Green Smoothie with Miner's Lettuce,
  106
Green Star, 103
Green Stinger, 78
Green Strawberry Drink, 125
Guacamole Spread, Probiotic, 93

Hallelujah Diet, 137, 138, 139
Hawaiian Hibiscus, 101
Heavy Metals Be Gone, 77
Herb Garden, 90
Herbs, 22, 23
Hibiscus, Hawaiian, 101
Honeydew melon
  Honeydew & Dandelion, 99
  Mellow Mallow, 110
Horseradish greens
  Spicy Green Soup, 86
  Spicy Sinus Cleaner, 77
Horsetail
  For the Brave, 76
Hot Stuff, 106
Hubbard, Dave, 139
Hydrochloric acid, 17

I Can't Believe It's Green Smoothie,
  67
Immune Booster, 91
Impeachmint!, 64
Iron, 9–10

Jackfruit
  Tooty Fruity, 100
Jim's Basic Basil, 87
Juicing, 27–30

Kale. *See also* Curly kale; Dinosaur
    kale
  Banacado, 114
  Basic Balance, 57

Kale, *continued*
Berry Blue Smoothie, 120
Coco-Tango, 119
Favorite Green Smoothie, 66
Fennel Soup, 87
Green Smoothie Monster, 73
Herb Garden, 90
Lovely Green Goodness, 62
Morning Glory, 89
One Tough Banana, 89
Peachy Keen Green, 102
The Pear-fect Smoothie, 107
Pink and Green, 61
Poochie's Gourmet Green Smoothie, 127
Rabbit Patch, 92
Satisfying Smoothie, 79
Soup Gazpacho, 82
Steven's Tropical Wigmore-Inspired Energy Smoothie, 105
Sun Green Pudding, 114
Turkish Grove, 69
Kent Mango Bliss, 108
Kiwis
For the Brave, 76
Green Caprice, 103
Green Jungle Jamboree, 76
Oh Bay-Beh Bay-Beh, 100
Rocket Fuel Smoothie, 60
Shelah's Tangy Pudding, 109
Sun Green Pudding, 114
Knotweed
Prickly Anticancer Recipe, 75
Resveratrol Elixir of Life, 76
Kulvinskas, Viktoras, 12

Lambsquarters
Black Sheep, 68
Fruity Weeds, 104
Hot Stuff, 106
Lambsquarters Omega Pudding, 112
Wild Melon Smoothie, 100
Lassi, Savory Cucumber, 87
The Laughing Gorilla, 119
Lee, Josephine, 138
Leeks
Immune Booster, 91
Lemon Pudding, 111
Lettuce. *See individual varieties*

Lewis, Wayne, 4
Limes
Mango-Lime Pudding, 109
O-Mega Aphrodisiac, 97
Spicy Green Soup, 86
Liver
Liver Lover, 88
World's Safest Liver Cleanser, 78
Lovely Green Goodness, 62
Love Potion, 65
Lowenfels, Jeff, 4
Luna Blanca, 133

Mâche
Chicken Scratch, 78
Malkmus, George, 137
Mallow *(Malva)*
Green Jungle Jamboree, 76
Mellow Mallow, 110
Oregano Tummy Soother, 82
Mangoes
Basic Balance, 57
Christmas in June, 69
Cilantro Sparkle, 113
Coco-Tango, 119
Dancing Dandelion Smoothie, 58
Dandy Lions, 74
Dent de Lion, 58
European Black Currant Smoothie, 60
Forest Full of Trees, 98
Frozen Mango Mint, 120
Goji Berry Enchantment, 63
Green Caprice, 103
Green Julius, 69
Green Smoothie with Miner's Lettuce, 106
Heavy Metals Be Gone, 77
Kent Mango Bliss, 108
The Laughing Gorilla, 119
Lemon Pudding, 111
Mango-Lime Pudding, 109
Mango Tarragon, 92
Mellow Mallow, 110
Midsummer, 75
Oh, My, What'd Ya Put in Here? I Can't Believe This Is Good for Me! Smoothie, 123
Pineapple Spice Cake, 70
Purple Teeth Masquerade, 123

Resveratrol Elixir of Life, 76
Revitalizing Energizer Smoothie, 98
Romintic Mango, 64
Savory Cucumber Lassi, 87
Sergei's Party in Your Mouth Green
  Smoothie, 72
Spinach Pudding, 117
Steven's Tropical Wigmore Inspired
  Energy Smoothie, 105
Stinging Nettle Green Smoothie, 80
Sunlight on Soil, 114
Tooty Fruity, 100
Tropical Green Smoothie, 65
Velvet Green Smoothie, 80
Wheat Grass-Hopper, 72
Manich, Clent, 135–50
McCollum, E. V., 32
Medallion Melon Smoothie, 59
Mediterranean Soup, 81
Mellow Cricket, 122
Mellow Mallow, 110
Memory Booster Brain Smoothie, 61
Midsummer, 75
Milk thistle
  Prickly Anticancer Recipe, 75
  World's Safest Liver Cleanser, 78
Miller, Gregory T., 28
Miner's lettuce
  Delicious Spring Green Smoothie,
    126
  Green Jungle Jamboree, 76
  Green Smoothie with Miner's
    Lettuce, 106
  Miner's Lettuce Smoothie, 120
  Vitamin C Master Combo, 77
Mint
  Fig Fantasy, 70
  Frozen Mango Mint, 120
  Impeachmint!, 64
  Pompous Persimmon Cocktail, 101
  Raspberry Guava Mint Swirl, 122
  Refreshing Cucumber Spinach, 91
  Romintic Mango, 64
  Sunlight on Soil, 114
  Today's Discovery, 104
Moerman, Daniel, 20
Morning Glory, 89
Morning Spark, 102
Morning Zing Smoothie, 57
Mulberry Magic, 122

Mustard greens
  Mustard Musketeer, 84
  Scarlet Honey Mustard Spread, 93
  Spicy Green Soup, 86
MyAfya, 134

Nectarines
  Citrus Sunlight, 70
  Coco-Tango, 119
  Love Potion, 65
  Red Green Smoothie, 71
Neighbor's Garden, 83
Nutritional deficiencies, 8–14

Oak leaf lettuce
  Gooseberry Crush, 62
Oh, My, What'd Ya Put in Here? I
    Can't Believe This Is Good for Me!
    Smoothie, 123
Oh Bay-Beh Bay-Beh, 100
O-Mega Aphrodisiac, 97
One Tough Banana, 89
Oranges
  Blueberry Zing, 109
  Christmas in June, 69
  Cilantro Sparkle, 113
  Colon Surprise Pudding, 113
  European Black Currant Smoothie,
    60
  Every Morning, 67
  Fruity Weeds, 104
  Green Julius, 69
  Green Monkey Face, 124
  Green Pudding, 108
  The Laughing Gorilla, 119
  Midsummer, 75
  Morning Glory, 89
  Orange Aid, 93
  Orange Zest, 94
  Red Bandit, 110
  Revitalizing Energizer Smoothie, 98
  Rocket Fuel Smoothie, 60
  Spinach Freshness, 124
Oregano
  Herb Garden, 90
  Oregano Tummy Soother, 82
Organic food, 48–49
Original Raw Family Smoothie
    Improved, 61
Otteby, Kim, 134

Oxalic acid, 34
Oxidation, 27–29

Papayas
Green Jungle Jamboree, 76
Papayavocado Pudding, 109
P-P-Papaya Smoothie, 59
Parsley
Apricot Nectar, 122
Bloody Mary, 106
Blueberry Zing, 109
Blue Skies Green Smoothie, 67
Cantaloupe Parsley Smoothie, 57
Celery Soup, 94
Citrus Sunlight, 70
Coconut Chameleon, 115
Colon Surprise Pudding, 113
Cool Summer Smoothie, 86
Double Green Smoothie, 74
Emerald Applesauce, 121
Garden Walk, 85
Green Julius, 69
Green Pudding, 108
Green Smoothie Monster, 73
Green Star, 103
Heavy Metals Be Gone, 77
Liver Lover, 88
Midsummer, 75
Parsley Passion Smoothie, 58
Purple Green Smoothie, 95
Raw Family Green Soup, 95
Red Smoothie, 71
Saskatoon Sunrise, 65
Summer Splendor Smoothie, 97
Sweet Parsley Smoothie, 62
Velvet Green Smoothie, 80
Party in Your Mouth Green Smoothie,
Sergei's, 72
Peaches
"Bitter Delight" Cocktail, 98
Coco-Tango, 119
Dancing Dandelion Smoothie, 58
Impeachmint!, 64
Morning Zing Smoothie, 57
Mulberry Magic, 122
Oh, My, What'd Ya Put in Here?
I Can't Believe This Is Good for
Me! Smoothie, 123
Peachy Keen Green, 102
Perfectly Peachy, 59

Purslane Green Smoothie, 79
Splendid Calendula, 110
Summer Splendor Smoothie, 97
Pears
Berry Blue Smoothie, 120
"Bitter Delight" Cocktail, 98
Bleh! "So Bland, Why Did I Try
This, But It's Growing on Me"
Smoothie, 99
Chicken Scratch, 78
Dent de Lion, 58
Double Green Smoothie, 74
Good Stuff, 68
Grandiose Grape Smoothie, 121
Green Pudding, 108
Green Smoothie Monster, 73
Green Star, 103
Green Strawberry Drink, 125
I Can't Believe It's Green Smoothie,
67
Kent Mango Bliss, 108
Lambsquarters Omega Pudding,
112
Liver Lover, 88
Lovely Green Goodness, 62
Memory Booster Brain Smoothie,
61
Miner's Lettuce Smoothie, 120
The Pear-fect Smoothie, 107
Pineapple Pudding Waltz, 117
Pink and Green, 61
Pompous Persimmon Cocktail, 101
Radical Radish, 90
Silly Cilantro, 102
Smoothie of Success, 121
Turkish Grove, 69
Valya's Green Pudding, 112
Vitamin C Master Combo, 77
What a Pair!, 89
Wild Green Pear, 103
World's Safest Liver Cleanser, 78
Peas
Neighbor's Garden, 83
Perfectly Peachy, 59
Persimmons
Persimmon Green Smoothie, 116
Persimmon Pudding, 107
Pompous Persimmon Cocktail, 101
Pets, green smoothies for, 41–44,
127–28

Phytonutrients, 32
Pineapple
  Greena Colada, 63
  Green Pudding, 108
  Hawaiian Hibiscus, 101
  Mellow Cricket, 122
  Morning Spark, 102
  Morning Zing Smoothie, 57
  Pineapple Pudding Waltz, 117
  Pineapple Spice Cake, 70
  Pineapple Spin, 121
  Sergei's Party in Your Mouth Green
    Smoothie, 72
  Shelah's Tangy Pudding, 109
  Steven's Tropical Wigmore-Inspired
    Energy Smoothie, 105
  Sweet Tart Smoothie, 104
  Thunderstorm Smoothie, 60
  Tropical Green Smoothie, 65
  Valya's Green Pudding, 112
Pineapple guava
  Raspberry Guava Mint Swirl, 122
  Smoothie of Success, 121
  Thunderstorm Smoothie, 60
Pine needles
  Forest Full of Trees, 98
Pink and Green, 61
Plantain, 35
  Plantain Skin Smoothie, 129
Plums
  For the Brave, 76
  Sea Buckthorn Rumba, 99
Poisonous plants, 23–24
Pomegranates
  Antioxidant Longevity Smoothie,
    105
Pompous Persimmon Cocktail, 101
Poochie's Gourmet Green Smoothie,
  127
Popsicles, Green Smoothie, 125
P-P-Papaya Smoothie, 59
Price, Weston, 12
Prickly Anticancer Recipe, 75
Prickly Pear Green-Go, 101
Probiotic Guacamole Spread, 93
Processed foods, consumption of,
  8–12
Protein, 31–32
Prunes
  Colon Surprise Pudding, 113

Puddings
  Applesauce, 108
  Avo-Coco Pudding, 111
  Banacado, 114
  Blueberry Zing, 109
  Cilantro Sparkle, 113
  Coconut Chameleon, 115
  Coconut Dream Pudding, 116
  Colon Surprise Pudding, 113
  Double Green Pudding, 117
  Dreamsicle Smoothie, 115
  Durian Green Pudding, 111
  Green Pudding, 108
  Kent Mango Bliss, 108
  Lambsquarters Omega Pudding,
    112
  Lemon Pudding, 111
  making, 107
  Mango-Lime Pudding, 109
  Mellow Mallow, 110
  Papayavocado Pudding, 109
  The Pear-fect Smoothie, 107
  Persimmon Green Smoothie, 116
  Pineapple Pudding Waltz, 117
  Recette des Champs Congelés,
    116
  Red Bandit, 110
  Shelah's Tangy Pudding, 109
  Simply Delicious Double-Green
    Pudding, 80
  Spinach Pudding, 117
  Splendid Calendula, 110
  Strawberry Crème, 112
  Sun Green Pudding, 114
  Sunlight on Soil, 114
  Sweet and Salty Star Pudding, 113
  Three-Course Meal, 115
  Valya's Green Pudding, 112
Pumpkin leaves
  Neighbor's Garden, 83
Purple Green Smoothie, 95
Purple Teeth Masquerade, 123
Purslane
  Lambsquarters Omega Pudding,
    112
  Memory Booster Brain Smoothie,
    61
  Midsummer, 75
  O-Mega Aphrodisiac, 97
  Purslane Green Smoothie, 79

Rabbit Patch, 92
Radish greens
  Radical Radish, 90
  Spicy Green Soup, 86
Radish sprouts
  Immune Booster, 91
Raisins
  Revolution-Evolution, 66
  Sun Green Pudding, 114
  Sunlight on Soil, 114
Raspberries
  Fruity Weeds, 104
  Perfectly Peachy, 59
  Raspberry Guava Mint Swirl, 122
  Sweet and Sour, 124
Raw Family Green Soup, 95
Raw food diet, 16, 151–57
Recette des Champs Congelés, 116
Red Bandit, 110
Red Green Smoothie, 71
Red leaf lettuce
  Recette des Champs Congelés, 116
  Red Green Smoothie, 71
  Rocket Fuel Smoothie, 60
Red Smoothie, 71
Refreshing Cucumber Spinach, 91
Resveratrol Elixir of Life, 76
Revitalizing Energizer Smoothie, 98
Revolution-Evolution, 66
Rocket Fuel Smoothie, 60
Roe, Daphne, 10
Romaine lettuce
  Apple Green Smoothie, 64
  Applesauce, 108
  Double Green Pudding, 117
  Good Stuff, 68
  The Laughing Gorilla, 119
  Medallion Melon Smoothie, 59
  Oh, My, What'd Ya Put in Here?
    I Can't Believe This Is Good for
    Me! Smoothie, 123
  Persimmon Green Smoothie, 116
  Raspberry Guava Mint Swirl, 122
  Romintic Mango, 64
  Sergei's Party in Your Mouth Green
    Smoothie, 72
  Strawberry Crème, 112
  Sweet and Sour, 124
  Three-Course Meal, 115
  Wicked Watermelon Smoothie, 59

Romintic Mango, 64
Rose petals
  Love Potion, 65

Saskatoon Sunrise, 65
Satisfying Smoothie, 79
Sauerkraut
  Probiotic Guacamole Spread, 93
Savory Basil Soup, 85
Savory Cucumber Lassi, 87
Savoy cabbage
  Savory Basil Soup, 85
Scarlet Honey Mustard Spread, 93
Sea Buckthorn Rumba, 99
Seeds, 4–5
Sergei's Party in Your Mouth Green
  Smoothie, 72
Shelah's Tangy Pudding, 109
Shelton, Herbert, 46
Shepard, Martha Hunter, 4
Silly Cilantro, 102
Simply Delicious Double-Green
  Pudding, 80
Sinus Cleaner, Spicy, 77
Skin Smoothie, Plantain, 129
Smoothie of Success, 121
Sorrel
  Love Potion, 65
  Vitamin C Master Combo, 77
Soups
  Celery Soup, 94
  Celery Zing Soup, 94
  Cucumber Dill-icious Soup, 82
  Fennel Soup, 87
  Mediterranean Soup, 81
  Mustard Musketeer, 84
  Orange Aid, 93
  Raw Family Green Soup, 95
  Savory Basil Soup, 85
  Soup Gazpacho, 82
  Spicy Green Soup, 86
  Sweet Soup, 95
  Thai Soup, 83
Spicy Green Soup, 86
Spicy Sinus Cleaner, 77
Spinach
  Andrea's Green Delight, 68
  Antioxidant Longevity Smoothie,
    105
  Christmas in June, 69

Clementine Citrus Circus, 123
Coco-nash Smoothie, 125
Daily Meal, 79
Double Green Pudding, 117
Durian Green Pudding, 111
Every Morning, 67
Fido's Dream, 128
Fig Fantasy, 70
Forest Full of Trees, 98
Garden Walk, 85
Greena Colada, 63
Green Julius, 69
Green Monkey Face, 124
Green Smoothie Popsicles!, 125
Impeachmint!, 64
Jim's Basic Basil, 87
Lemon Pudding, 111
Mediterranean Soup, 81
Mulberry Magic, 122
oxalic acid in, 34
Papayavocado Pudding, 109
Persimmon Pudding, 107
Pineapple Spin, 121
P-P-Papaya Smoothie, 59
Probiotic Guacamole Spread, 93
Refreshing Cucumber Spinach, 91
Smoothie of Success, 121
Spicy Green Soup, 86
Spinach Cold Buster, 92
Spinach Freshness, 124
Spinach Pudding, 117
Springtime Douglas Fir Smoothie,
     105
Sunlight on Soil, 114
Sweet and Sour, 124
Three-Course Meal, 115
Tropical Green Smoothie, 65
Winter Green Smoothie, 63, 72
Splendid Calendula, 110
Spreads
   Probiotic Guacamole Spread, 93
   Scarlet Honey Mustard Spread, 93
Springtime Douglas Fir Smoothie, 105
Sprouts, 22–23. See also individual
     sprouts
Squash leaves
   Neighbor's Garden, 83
Standard American Diet (SAD), 16
Star fruit
   Sweet and Salty Star Pudding, 113

Thunderstorm Smoothie, 60
Steven's Tropical Wigmore-Inspired
     Energy Smoothie, 105
Stinging nettles
   Green Stinger, 78
   Heavy Metals Be Gone, 77
   Stinging Nettle Green Smoothie, 80
Stomach acid test, 17
Stool, green, 36
Strawberries
   Coconut Chameleon, 115
   Double Green Pudding, 117
   Dreamsicle Smoothie, 115
   Every Morning, 67
   Forest Full of Trees, 98
   Frozen Mango Mint, 120
   Green Caprice, 103
   Green Strawberry Drink, 125
   Original Raw Family Smoothie
     Improved, 61
   Pink and Green, 61
   Prickly Anticancer Recipe, 75
   Red Green Smoothie, 71
   Revitalizing Energizer Smoothie, 98
   Smoothie of Success, 121
   Spinach Freshness, 124
   Strawberry Crème, 112
Summer Splendor Smoothie, 97
Summertime Smoothie, 71
Sunflower sprouts
   Green Star, 103
   Mellow Cricket, 122
   Steven's Tropical Wigmore-Inspired
     Energy Smoothie, 105
Sun Green Pudding, 114
Sunlight on Soil, 114
Sweet and Salty Star Pudding, 113
Sweet and Sour, 124
Sweet Parsley Smoothie, 62
Sweet Soup, 95
Sweet Tart Smoothie, 104

Tangelos
   Citrus Sunlight, 70
   Yummerific, 66
Tangerines
   Goji Berry Enchantment, 63
Thai Soup, 83
Three-Course Meal, 115
Thunderstorm Smoothie, 60

Today's Discovery, 104
Tomatoes
  All Kinds of Peppers and Tomatoes, 84
  Bloody Mary, 106
  Celery Soup, 94
  Daily Meal, 79
  Garden Walk, 85
  Herb Garden, 90
  I Can't Believe It's Green Smoothie, 67
  Jim's Basic Basil, 87
  Neighbor's Garden, 83
  Rabbit Patch, 92
  Savory Basil Soup, 85
  Soup Gazpacho, 82
  Spicy Green Soup, 86
  Spicy Sinus Cleaner, 77
  Victoria's Favorite Dark Green, 73
Tooty Fruity, 100
Tropical Green Smoothie, 65
Tummy Soother, Oregano, 82
Turkish Grove, 69
Turnip greens
  Neighbor's Garden, 83

Valya's Green Pudding, 112
Vegetables. *See also individual vegetables*
  food combining and, 45–46
  organic, 48–49
  starchy, 46, 48
Velvet Green Smoothie, 80
Vetrano, Vivian, 35
Victoria's Favorite Dark Green, 73

Vitamin C Master Combo, 77
Vitamins
  B12, 35
  C, 10, 77
  K, 12–14

Watercress
  Spicy Green Soup, 86
  Spicy Sinus Cleaner, 77
Watermelon
  Aphrodisiac Cocktail, 100
  Love Potion, 65
  O-Mega Aphrodisiac, 97
  Rabbit Patch, 92
  Wicked Watermelon Smoothie, 59
Weeds, 22, 24, 35
Weight loss, 135–50
Wells, Anand, 132
What a Pair!, 89
Wheatgrass, 32
  Fluffy's Delight, 128
  Wheat Grass-Hopper, 72
Wicked Watermelon Smoothie, 59
Wigmore, Anne, 46
Wild greens, 22, 24, 35
  Wild Green Pear, 103
Wild Melon Smoothie, 100
Winter Green Smoothie, 63, 72
World's Safest Liver Cleanser, 78

Yummerific, 66

Zucchini
  Bok Choy Joy, 88
  Liver Lover, 88
  Neighbor's Garden, 83

ACKNOWLEDGMENTS

I acknowledge all the people who shared their favorite green smoothie recipes with the world.

I am grateful to my family for their endless patience, love, and support while I was working on this book.

My heart goes out to all the friends who volunteered to spend many hours editing my manuscript: Aletha Nowitzky, Vanessa Nowitzky, Bridget Wolf, and Leslie DeLorean.

I thank Robert Petetit for his lovely photographs.

I greatly appreciate Dr. Miven Donato, Clent Manich, and Gabrielle Chavez for their valuable contributions to this book.

With Green Love,
Victoria